This book belongs to

....

CONTENTS

How to Use this Book 4

BEFORE YOU WERE BORN **6**
Mummy and Daddy 8
Before You Were Born 10

YOUR FIRST YEAR **14**
Your Birth 16
All About You 20
On the Day You Were Born 22
This is Our Family 24
Our Family Tree 28
Your First Week 32
Your First Visitors 36
We Celebrated Your Arrival 40
'Any-Day' Records and Photos 42
Things We Like to Do Together 54
Bathtime 58
Your Bedtime Routine 60
Your Friends 62
Reflections 66
Your First Christmas 68
Your First Holiday 72
Occasions to Remember 74
You and Your Food 78
Your First Birthday 80

YOUR SECOND YEAR **82**
Now You Are One ... 84
'Any-Day' Records and Photos 86
Places You Like to Visit 98
Your Friends 100
Things We Like to Do Together 102
Messy Mealtimes 106
Your Bedtime Routine 108
Reflections 110
Your Second Christmas 112
Occasions to Remember 114
Holidays 118
Your Second Birthday 120

YOUR THIRD YEAR   122

Now You Are Two …   124
'Any-Day' Records and Photos   126
Places You Like to Visit   138
Your Friends   140
Things We Like to Do Together   144
Reflections   148
Your Favourite Recipes   150
Your Bedtime Routine   154
Your Third Christmas   156
Occasions to Remember   158
Holidays   162
Your Third Birthday   164

HOW YOU GREW AND CHANGED   166

Your Development   168
Your Health   172
Your Tooth Chart   174
Your Milestones   176
What You Said and When   180
Your First Masterpieces   182
Here Comes Trouble   186
Your First Day at Nursery   188
Your Unique Firsts   190
Your Life So Far …   194
Looking Back …   198
Messages from Your Family   200

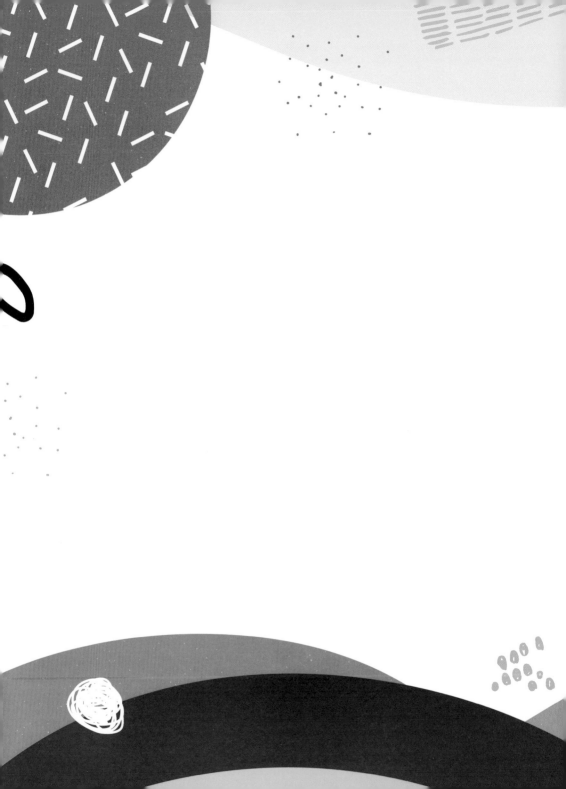

HOW TO USE THIS BOOK

The *Baby Book* covers the period from just before the birth to your child's third birthday. There is space for reflecting and making notes of 'firsts' and your daily routine, as well as room for sticking in photographs. There is also a pocket at the back of the book for preserving keepsakes, clippings or drawings.

As your child gets older it can be fun to look back through the book, sharing memories, looking at photos and making new entries together. Remember that it is often the everyday routine activities that we forget about and older children always love to hear about what they used to do when they were little, so write about the ordinary as well as the special days. You can encourage grandparents, aunts, uncles and even siblings to contribute too.

Most important of all, this is your record of your baby's first years so enter whatever is important to you and what you think you will want to remember. Scribble notes, stuff in pictures, it doesn't have to look beautiful and you don't have to do it every day. Just have fun with it, and tell the story of these first years together, filling it in when you can.

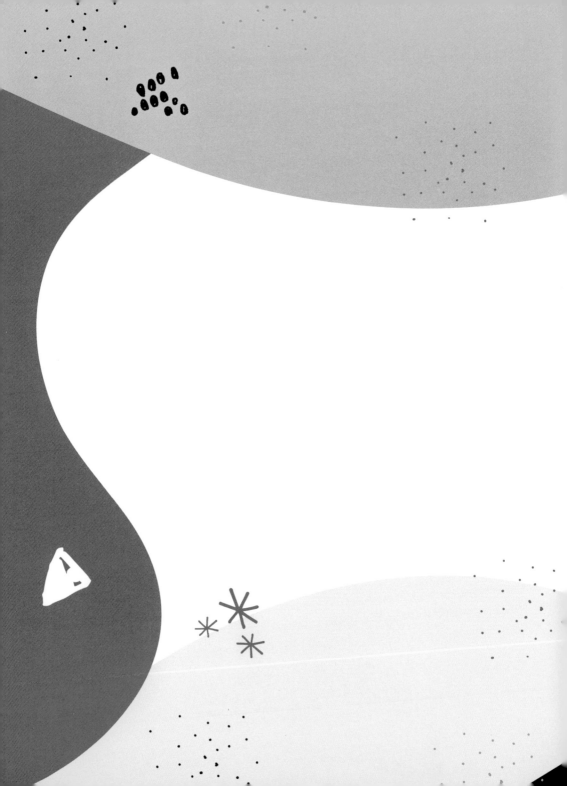

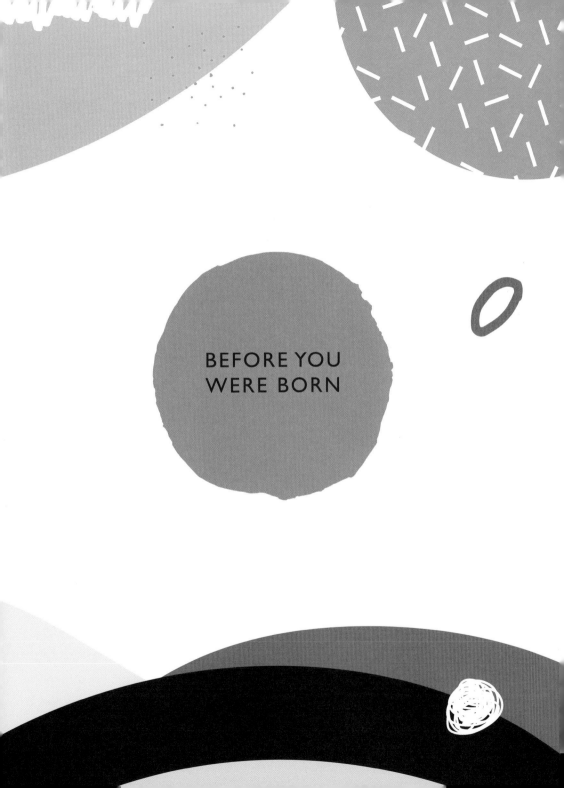

BEFORE YOU
WERE BORN

MUMMY

FULL NAME:

NICKNAME:

DATE OF BIRTH:

BORN IN (LOCATION):

MUMMY'S JOB:

MUMMY'S FAVOURITE SONG:

MUMMY'S FAVOURITE HOBBY:

MUMMY'S FAVOURITE FOOD:

MUMMY

DATE:

DADDY

FULL NAME:

NICKNAME:

DATE OF BIRTH:

BORN IN (LOCATION):

DADDY'S JOB:

DADDY'S FAVOURITE SONG:

DADDY'S FAVOURITE HOBBY:

DADDY'S FAVOURITE FOOD:

DADDY

DATE:

BEFORE YOU WERE BORN

WE FOUND OUT ABOUT YOU ON:

....

....

YOU WERE DUE TO BE BORN ON:

....

....

A STORY FROM MUMMY'S PREGNANCY:

....

....

....

....

....

....

....

....

MUMMY'S FAVOURITE FOOD/CRAVINGS WHILE PREGNANT:

....

....

....

....

YOUR BABY SHOWER WAS ON:

....

....

....

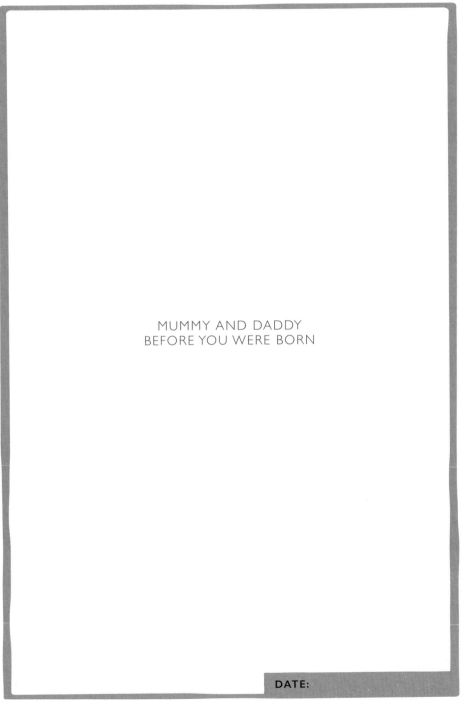

MUMMY AND DADDY
BEFORE YOU WERE BORN

DATE:

BEFORE YOU WERE BORN OUR NICKNAME FOR YOU WAS:

....
....

THESE WERE SOME OF THE NAMES WE THOUGHT ABOUT CALLING YOU:

....
....
....
....
....
....
....
....
....

WHAT WE WISH FOR YOU:

....
....
....
....
....
....
....
....
....
....
....
....

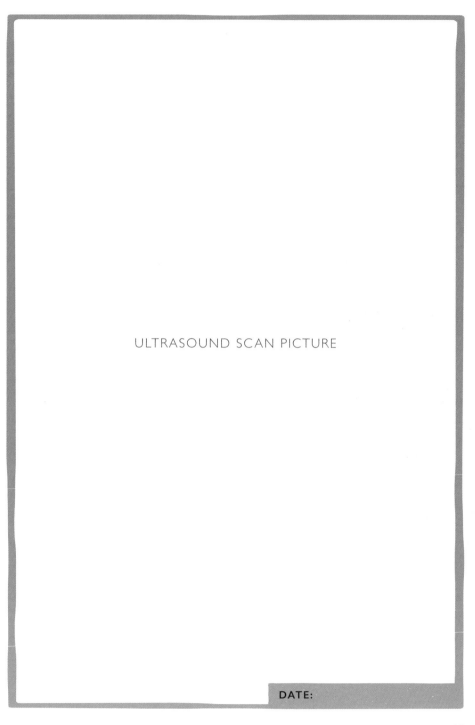

ULTRASOUND SCAN PICTURE

DATE:

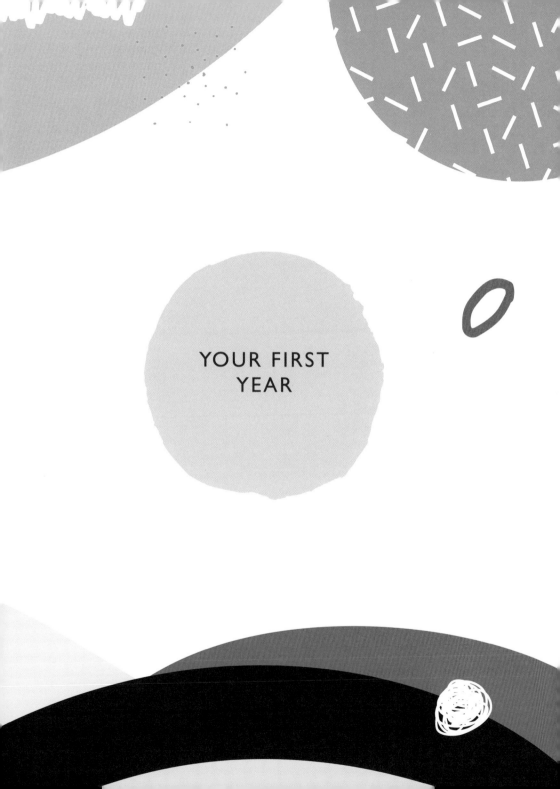

YOUR FIRST
YEAR

YOUR BIRTH

NAME:

WAS BORN ON:

AT (PLACE):

AT (TIME):

PRESENT AT THE BIRTH WERE:

MIDWIFE:

DOCTOR:

FIRST PICTURES OF YOU

DATE:

FIRST PICTURES OF YOU

DATE:

YOUR BIRTH

REFLECTIONS:

WHEN YOU WERE BORN EVERYONE HAD AN OPINION ABOUT WHOM YOU
LOOKED LIKE:

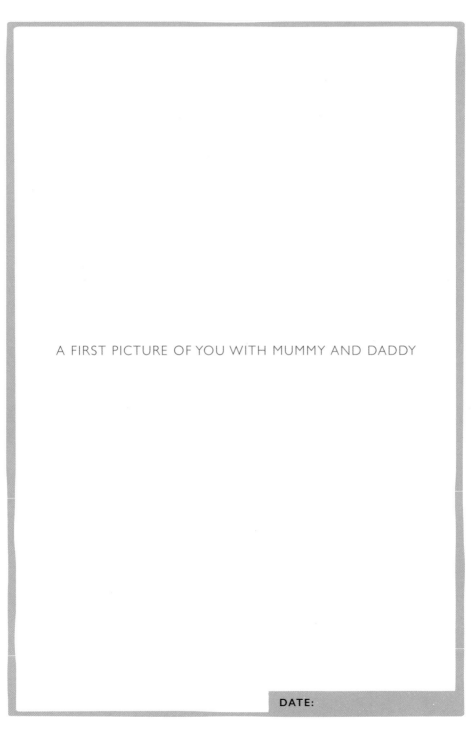

A FIRST PICTURE OF YOU WITH MUMMY AND DADDY

DATE:

ALL ABOUT YOU

WEIGHT:

LENGTH:

HEAD CIRCUMFERENCE:

EYE COLOUR:

HAIR TYPE AND COLOUR:

THIS IS AN IMPRINT OF YOUR HAND...

IMPRINT OF YOUR HAND

DATE:

STAR SIGN:

CHINESE ZODIAC ANIMAL:

YOU SHARE YOUR BIRTHDAY WITH (ANY FAMILY MEMBER OR
FAMOUS PEOPLE):

THIS IS AN IMPRINT OF YOUR FOOT...

IMPRINT OF YOUR FOOT

DATE:

ON THE DAY YOU WERE BORN

THE HEADLINES WERE:

THE WEATHER WAS:

POPULAR SONGS WERE:

THE LEADER OF THE GOVERNMENT, & THE POLITICAL PARTY IN POWER, WAS:

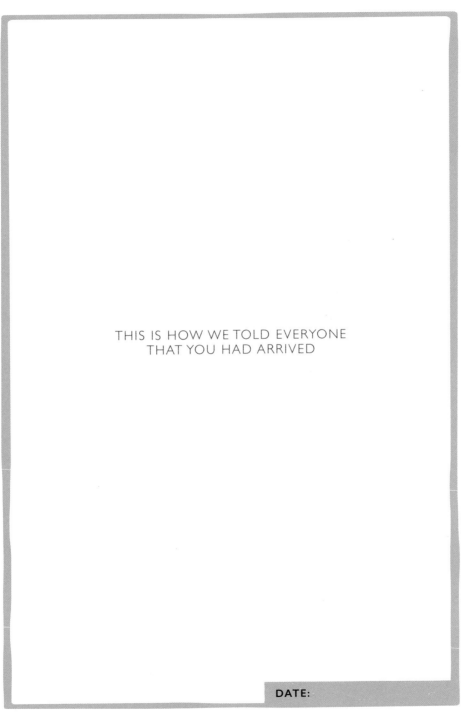

THIS IS HOW WE TOLD EVERYONE
THAT YOU HAD ARRIVED

DATE:

Describe and list the members of your immediate family (including pets!), and then take a moment to write about the family home.

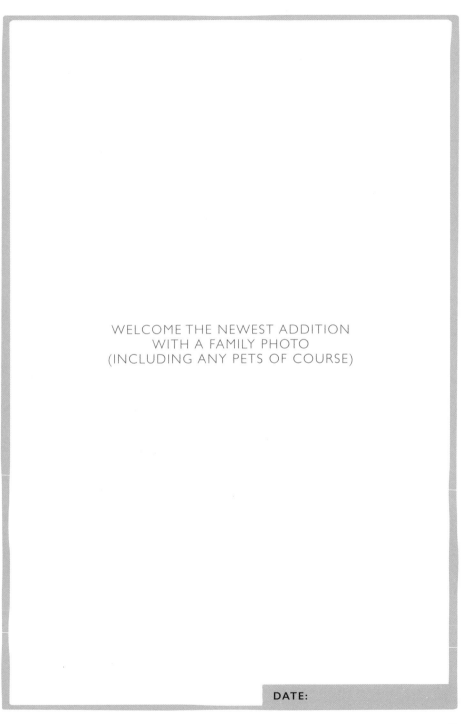

WELCOME THE NEWEST ADDITION
WITH A FAMILY PHOTO
(INCLUDING ANY PETS OF COURSE)

DATE:

THIS IS OUR FAMILY

WE LIVE AT:

WE HAVE LIVED HERE FOR:

OUR NEIGHBOURS ARE:

YOUR FIRST BEDROOM WAS DECORATED WITH:

OUR HOME

DATE:

OUR GARDEN

DATE:

OUR FAMILY TREE

Record as much detail as you can about family members: their full names, where they were born and dates such as birth, marriage and death.

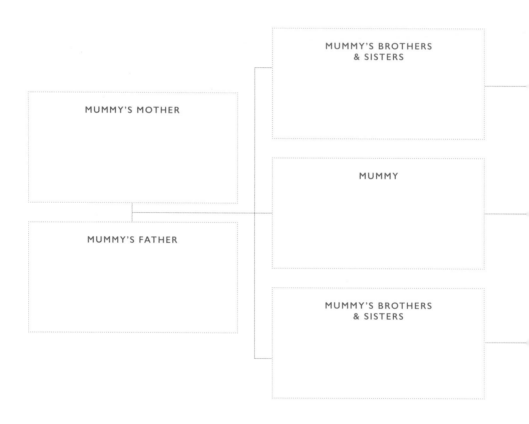

MUMMY'S BROTHERS & SISTERS

MUMMY'S MOTHER

MUMMY

MUMMY'S FATHER

MUMMY'S BROTHERS & SISTERS

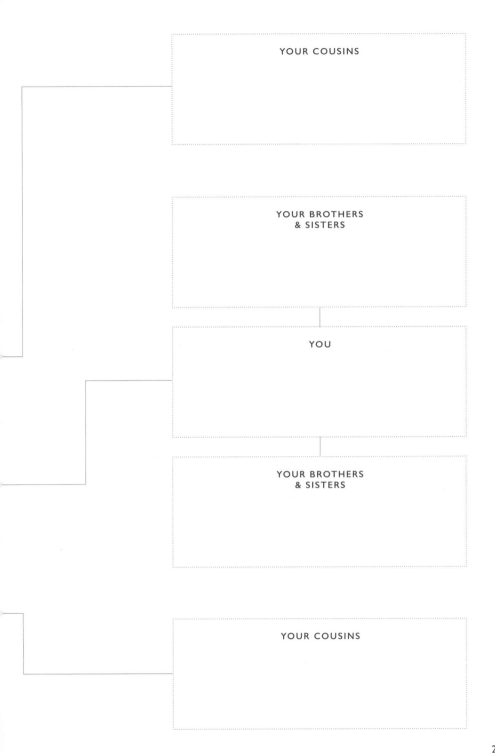

YOUR COUSINS

YOUR BROTHERS
& SISTERS

YOU

YOUR BROTHERS
& SISTERS

YOUR COUSINS

Record as much detail as you can about family members: their full names, where they were born and dates such as birth, marriage and death.

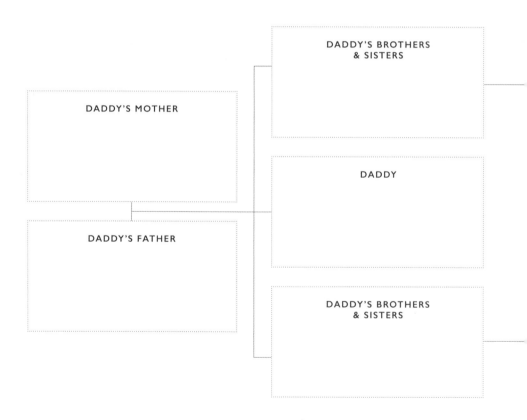

YOUR COUSINS

OTHER IMPORTANT PEOPLE IN OUR FAMILY

YOUR COUSINS

YOUR FIRST WEEK

The first week often disappears in a blur of sleepless nights and seemingly endless feeds and changes. Make a note here of where it was spent, what you did as a family, and how baby ate and slept. Record baby's moods and your own thoughts and feelings, along with those of other members of the family, including any brothers and sisters.

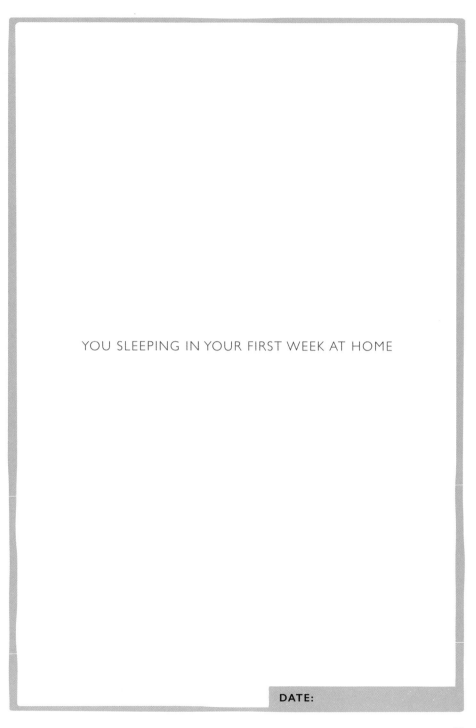

YOU SLEEPING IN YOUR FIRST WEEK AT HOME

DATE:

YOUR FIRST WEEK

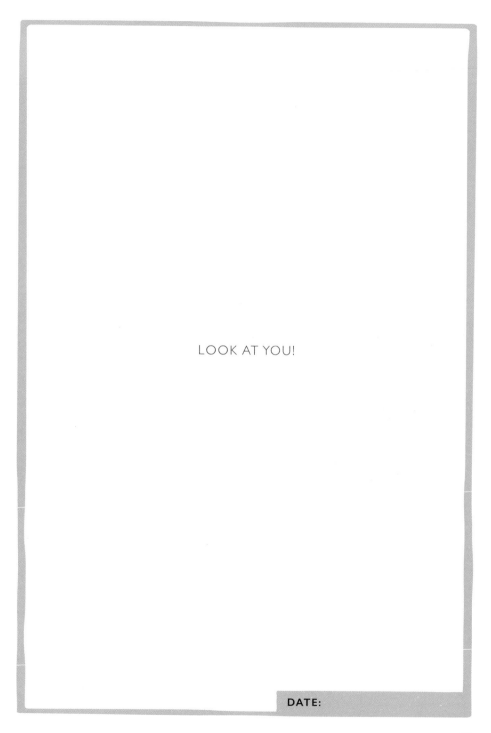

LOOK AT YOU!

DATE:

YOUR FIRST VISITORS

These are some of the friends and family who visited and brought you presents and cards:

EVERYONE WANTS THEIR
PHOTOGRAPH TAKEN WITH YOU

YOUR FIRST VISITORS

These are some of the friends and family who visited and brought you presents and cards:

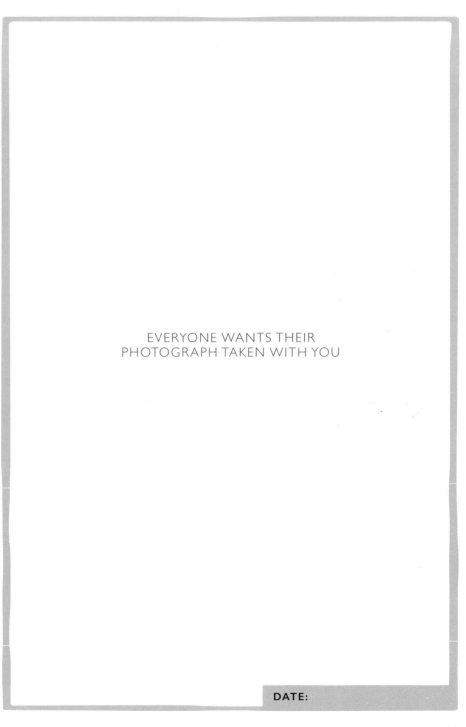

EVERYONE WANTS THEIR
PHOTOGRAPH TAKEN WITH YOU

DATE:

WE CELEBRATED YOUR ARRIVAL

ON:

AT:

GODPARENTS/SPONSORS:

GUESTS:

FRIENDS AND FAMILY WHO COULD NOT JOIN US ON THE DAY INCLUDED:

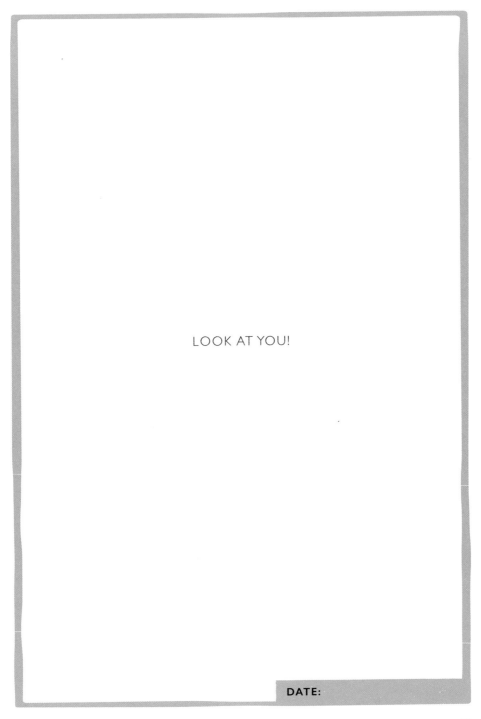

LOOK AT YOU!

DATE:

'ANY-DAY' RECORDS AND PHOTOS

AGE:

DATE:

YOU WAKE UP AT:

YOU GET UP AT:

YOU HAVE A NAP AT:

YOUR BEDTIME IS:

YOU ARE FED AT:

OBSERVATIONS:

YOU LIKE:

YOU DON'T LIKE:

MINI MILESTONES:

YOUR FAVOURITE THINGS ARE:

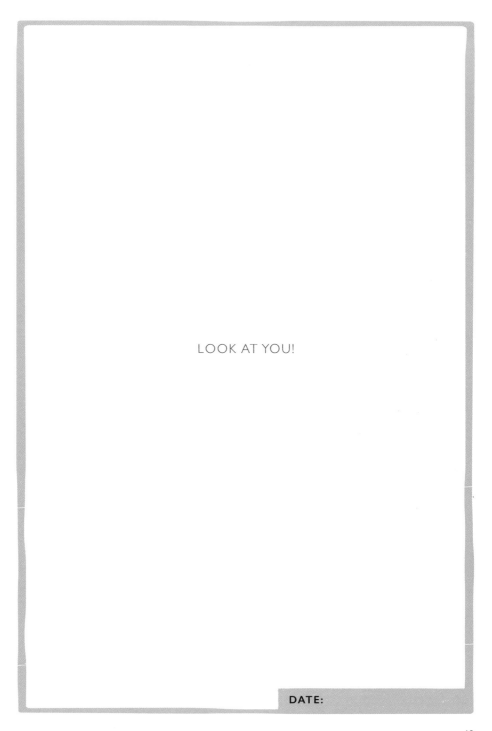

LOOK AT YOU!

DATE:

'ANY-DAY' RECORDS AND PHOTOS

AGE:

DATE:

YOU WAKE UP AT:

YOU GET UP AT:

YOU HAVE A NAP AT:

YOUR BEDTIME IS:

YOU ARE FED AT:

OBSERVATIONS:

YOU LIKE:

YOU DON'T LIKE:

MINI MILESTONES:

YOUR FAVOURITE THINGS ARE:

AGE:

DATE:

YOU WAKE UP AT:

YOU GET UP AT:

YOU HAVE A NAP AT:

YOUR BEDTIME IS:

YOU ARE FED AT:

OBSERVATIONS:

YOU LIKE:

YOU DON'T LIKE:

MINI MILESTONES:

YOUR FAVOURITE THINGS ARE:

'ANY-DAY' RECORDS AND PHOTOS

AGE:

DATE:

YOU WAKE UP AT:

YOU GET UP AT:

YOU HAVE A NAP AT:

YOUR BEDTIME IS:

YOU ARE FED AT:

OBSERVATIONS:

YOU LIKE:

YOU DON'T LIKE:

MINI MILESTONES:

YOUR FAVOURITE THINGS ARE:

AGE:

DATE:

YOU WAKE UP AT:

YOU GET UP AT:

YOU HAVE A NAP AT:

YOUR BEDTIME IS:

YOU ARE FED AT:

OBSERVATIONS:

YOU LIKE:

YOU DON'T LIKE:

MINI MILESTONES:

YOUR FAVOURITE THINGS ARE:

'ANY-DAY' RECORDS AND PHOTOS

AGE:

DATE:

YOU WAKE UP AT:

YOU GET UP AT:

YOU HAVE A NAP AT:

YOUR BEDTIME IS:

YOU ARE FED AT:

OBSERVATIONS:

YOU LIKE:

YOU DON'T LIKE:

MINI MILESTONES:

YOUR FAVOURITE THINGS ARE:

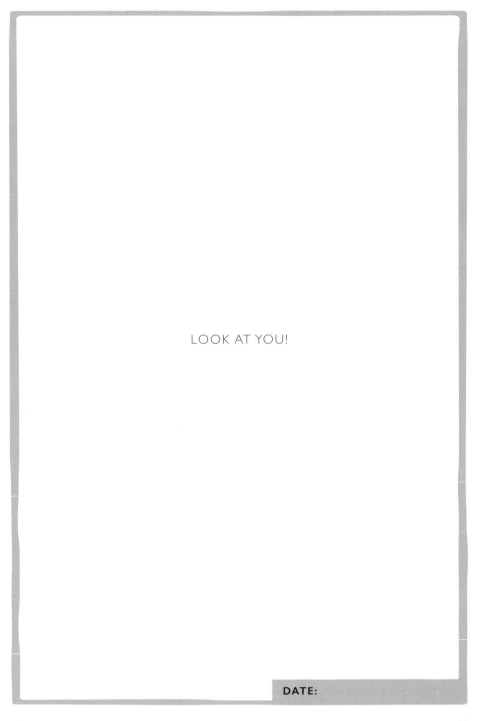

LOOK AT YOU!

DATE:

AGE:

DATE:

YOU WAKE UP AT:

YOU GET UP AT:

YOU HAVE A NAP AT:

YOUR BEDTIME IS:

YOU ARE FED AT:

OBSERVATIONS:

YOU LIKE:

YOU DON'T LIKE:

MINI MILESTONES:

YOUR FAVOURITE THINGS ARE:

AGE:

DATE:

YOU WAKE UP AT:

YOU GET UP AT:

YOU HAVE A NAP AT:

YOUR BEDTIME IS:

YOU ARE FED AT:

OBSERVATIONS:

YOU LIKE:

YOU DON'T LIKE:

MINI MILESTONES:

YOUR FAVOURITE THINGS ARE:

'ANY-DAY' RECORDS AND PHOTOS

AGE:

DATE:

YOU WAKE UP AT:

YOU GET UP AT:

YOU HAVE A NAP AT:

YOUR BEDTIME IS:

YOU ARE FED AT:

OBSERVATIONS:

YOU LIKE:

YOU DON'T LIKE:

MINI MILESTONES:

YOUR FAVOURITE THINGS ARE:

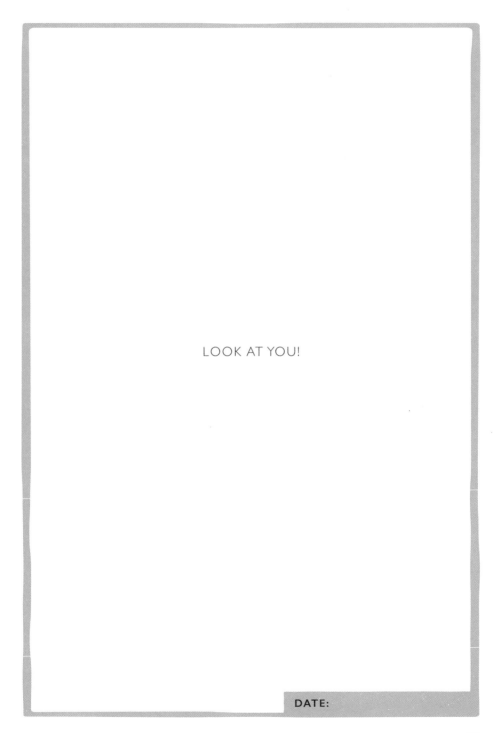

LOOK AT YOU!

DATE:

THINGS WE LIKE TO DO TOGETHER

What do you and your baby like to do together? Do you have favourite songs or games? Perhaps you like to go to the park or swimming. It's often the everyday activities that we forget so easily, but these are the activities that forge our relationship and which shape your baby's life, so record them here to share together later.

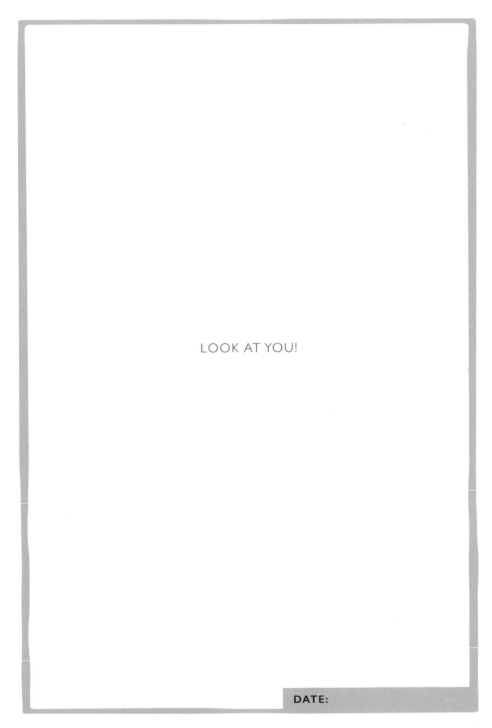

LOOK AT YOU!

DATE:

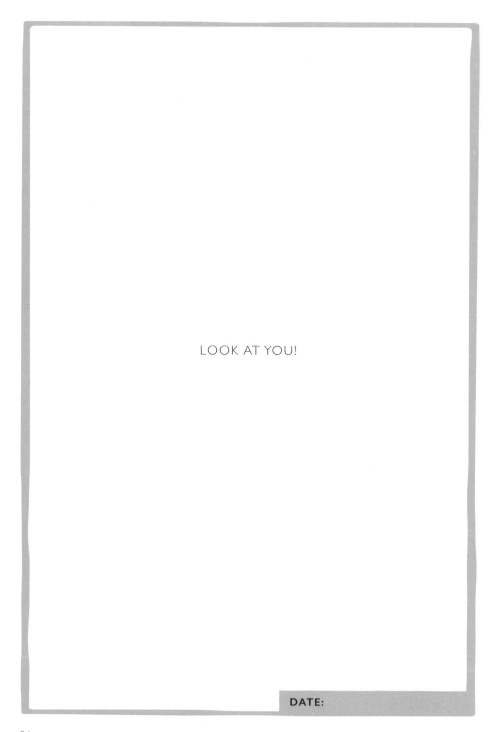

LOOK AT YOU!

DATE:

THINGS WE LIKE TO DO TOGETHER

BATHTIME

WHAT YOU LIKE BEST ABOUT BATHTIME IS:

WHAT YOU HATE MOST ABOUT BATHTIME IS:

YOUR FAVOURITE BATHTIME TOYS AND GAMES ARE:

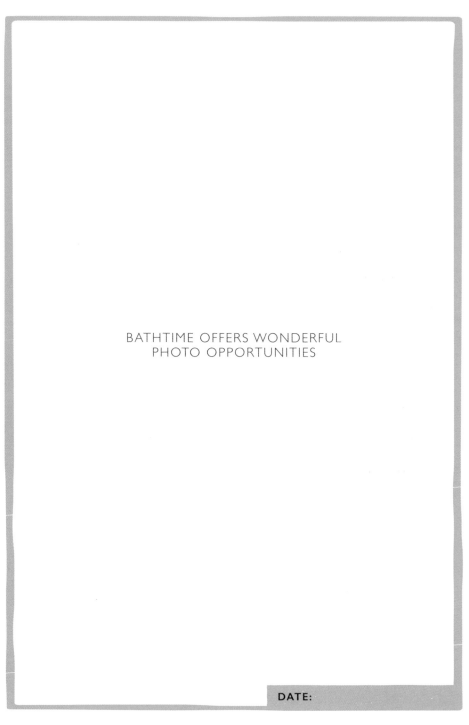

BATHTIME OFFERS WONDERFUL
PHOTO OPPORTUNITIES

DATE:

YOUR BEDTIME ROUTINE

YOU GO TO SLEEP AT:

....

....

BEFORE YOU GO TO SLEEP YOU LIKE:

....

....

....

....

....

....

....

YOUR FAVOURITE LULLABIES AND BOOKS AT BEDTIME ARE:

....

....

....

....

....

....

OTHER COMMENTS:

....

....

....

....

....

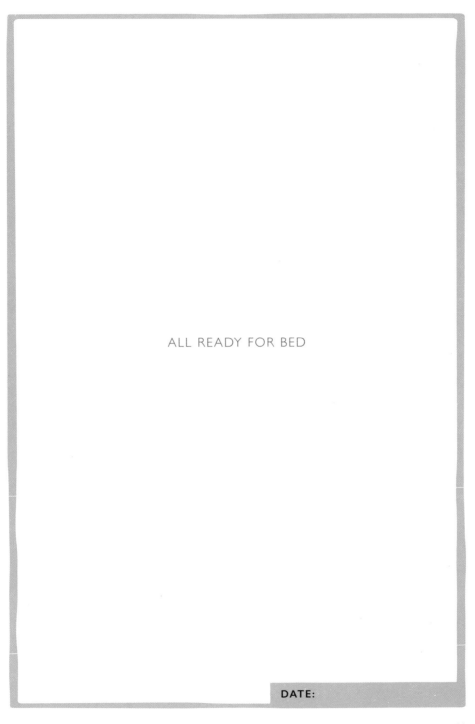

ALL READY FOR BED

DATE:

YOUR FRIENDS

Making friends and learning to play together is part of growing up. Record your baby's early friendships in words and pictures.

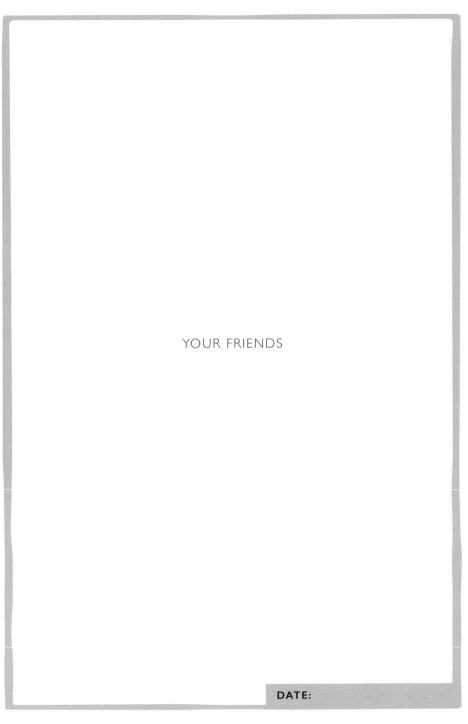

YOUR FRIENDS

DATE:

YOUR FRIENDS

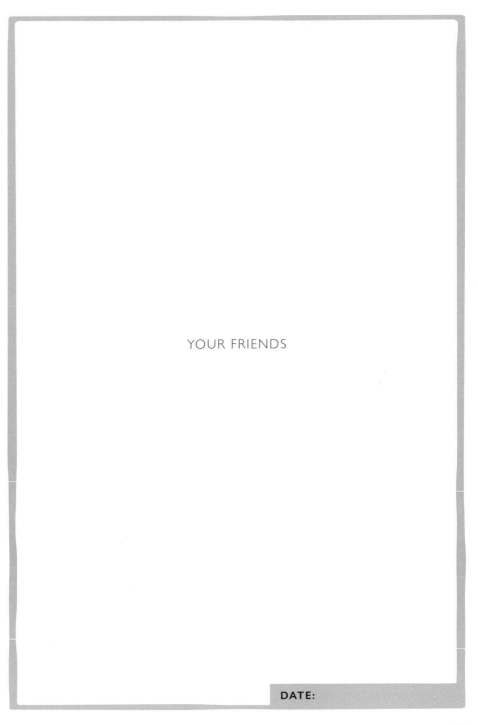

YOUR FRIENDS

REFLECTIONS

It's easy to get lost in the busyness of everyday living, so why not take some time to reflect back over these first months together; your favourite moments and your difficult times too. Record what you have learned about yourself and each other, as well as your baby.

YOUR FIRST CHRISTMAS

AGE:

....

....

WE SPENT CHRISTMAS EVE AT:

....

WITH:

....

....

....

....

WE SPENT CHRISTMAS DAY AT:

....

WITH:

....

....

....

....

YOUR CHRISTMAS OUTFIT WAS:

....

....

....

....

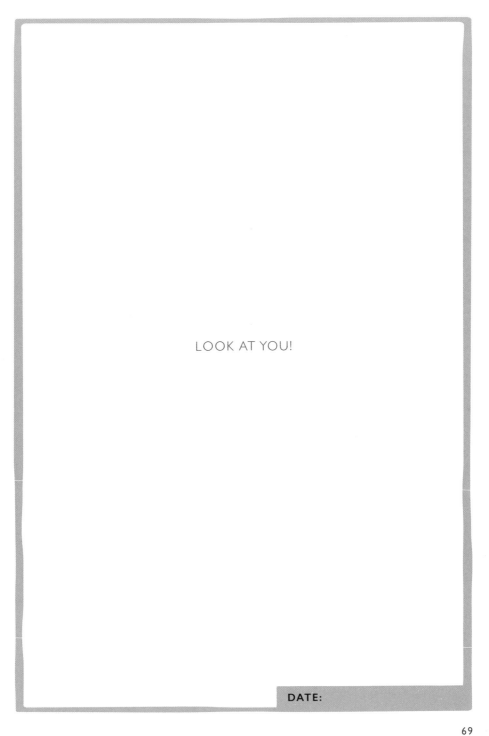

LOOK AT YOU!

DATE:

YOUR FIRST CHRISTMAS

YOU ATE:

....

....

....

....

....

....

....

YOU RECEIVED LOTS OF PRESENTS INCLUDING:

....

....

....

....

....

....

....

YOU ENJOYED:

....

....

....

....

....

....

....

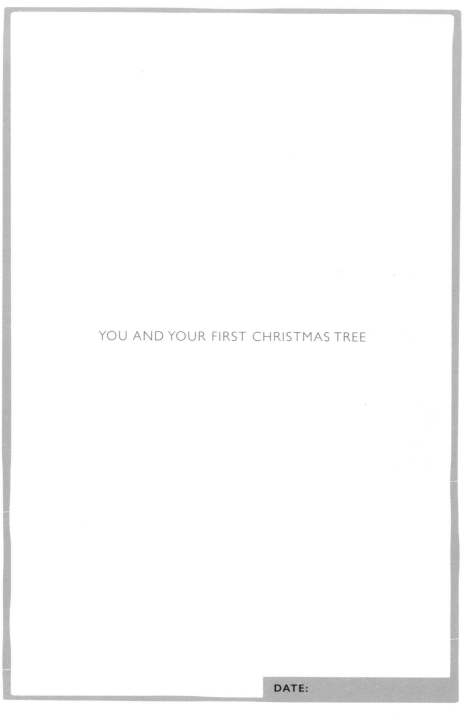

YOU AND YOUR FIRST CHRISTMAS TREE

YOUR FIRST HOLIDAY

AGE:

WE WENT TO:

ON:

FOR:

YOUR FAVOURITE THING ABOUT THE HOLIDAY WAS:

YOU LIKED:

YOU DIDN'T LIKE:

REFLECTIONS:

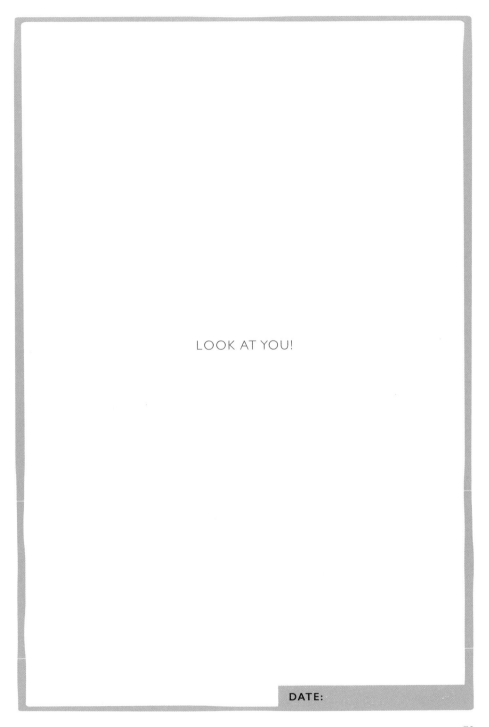

LOOK AT YOU!

DATE:

Every year has memorable events, from family weddings and births to christenings or naming ceremonies. Use these pages to record what was celebrated when, who was there and what was special about it.

OCCASION:
....

DATE:
....

WHO WAS THERE:
....

....

....

....

....

MEMORIES OF THE DAY:
....

....

....

....

....

....

....

....

OCCASION:

DATE:

WHO WAS THERE:

MEMORIES OF THE DAY:

OCCASIONS TO REMEMBER

OCCASION:

DATE:

WHO WAS THERE:

MEMORIES OF THE DAY:

OCCASION:

DATE:

WHO WAS THERE:

MEMORIES OF THE DAY:

YOU AND YOUR FOOD

YOU WERE WEANED ON:

YOUR FIRST FINGER FOOD WAS:

YOUR FIRST SOLIDS WERE:

YOUR FIRST PROPER MEALS WERE:

YOU FIRST USED A BEAKER FOR:

YOU FIRST FED YOURSELF ON:

YOU FIRST USED CUTLERY ON:

DATE TRIED:				
PURÉED FOOD Write type of food and your baby's reaction				

DATE TRIED:				
FINGER FOOD Write type of food and your baby's reaction				

DATE TRIED:				
SOLID FOOD Write type of food and your baby's reaction				

YOUR FIRST BIRTHDAY

WAS SPENT AT:

....

....

....

....

YOU WERE GIVEN:

....

....

....

....

....

....

YOUR CAKE WAS:

....

....

....

....

....

ON YOUR BIRTHDAY WE:

....

....

....

....

....

....

....

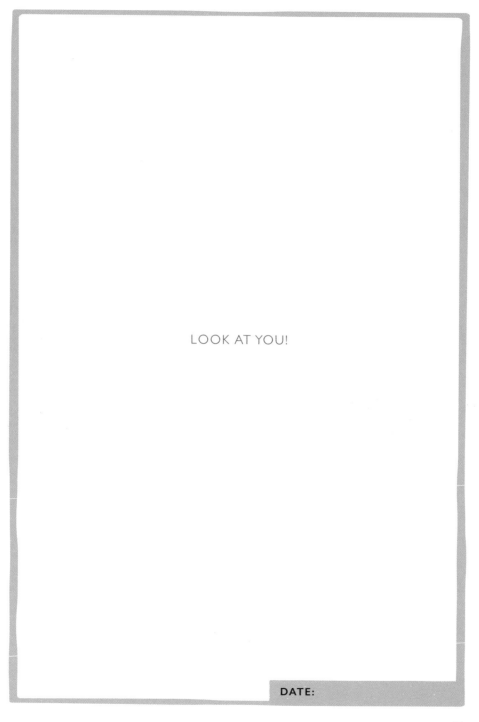

LOOK AT YOU!

DATE:

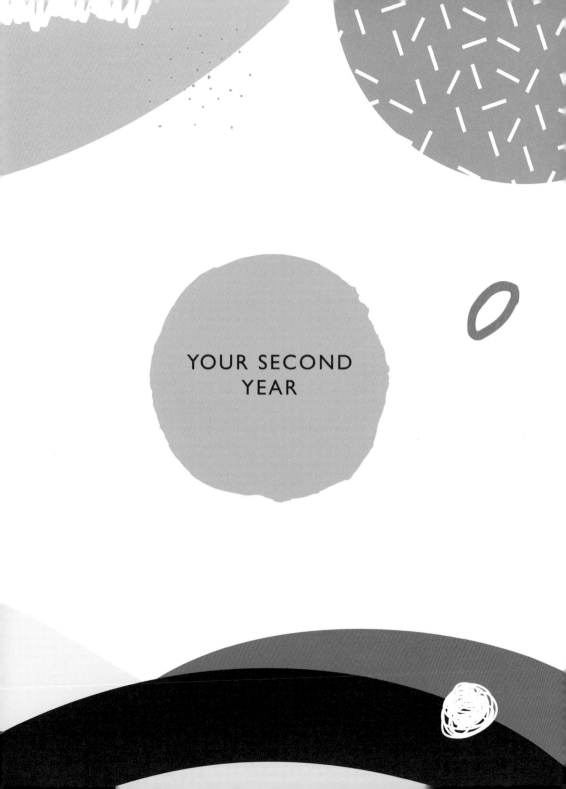

YOUR SECOND
YEAR

NOW YOU ARE ONE ...

YOU ARE: CMS/INS TALL

YOU WEIGH: KGS/LBS

YOU CAN:

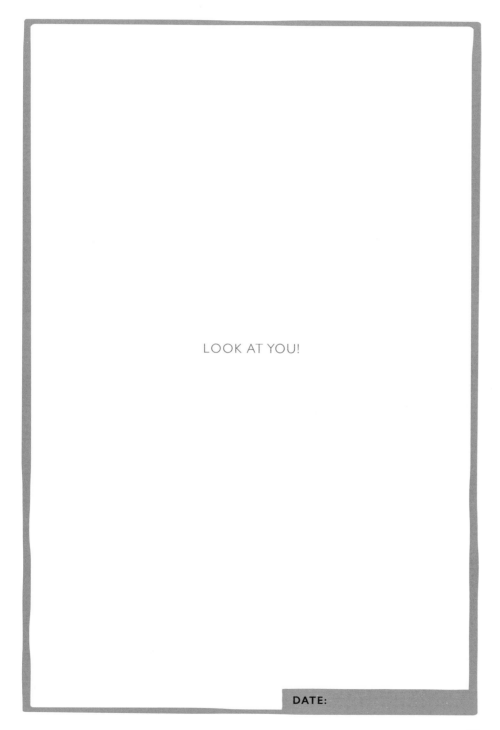

LOOK AT YOU!

DATE:

AGE:

DATE:

YOU WAKE UP AT:

YOU GET UP AT:

YOU HAVE A NAP AT:

YOUR BEDTIME IS:

YOU ARE FED AT:

MINI MILESTONES:

YOU LIKE:

YOU DON'T LIKE:

YOUR FAVOURITE GAMES AND TOYS ARE:

YOUR FAVOURITE SONGS AND RHYMES ARE:

YOUR FAVOURITE STORIES ARE:

YOUR FAVOURITE THINGS ARE:

AGE:

DATE:

YOU WAKE UP AT:

YOU GET UP AT:

YOU HAVE A NAP AT:

YOUR BEDTIME IS:

YOU ARE FED AT:

MINI MILESTONES:

YOU LIKE:

YOU DON'T LIKE:

YOUR FAVOURITE GAMES AND TOYS ARE:

YOUR FAVOURITE SONGS AND RHYMES ARE:

YOUR FAVOURITE STORIES ARE:

YOUR FAVOURITE THINGS ARE:

'ANY-DAY' RECORDS AND PHOTOS

AGE:

DATE:

YOU WAKE UP AT:

YOU GET UP AT:

YOU HAVE A NAP AT:

YOUR BEDTIME IS:

YOU ARE FED AT:

MINI MILESTONES:

YOU LIKE:

YOU DON'T LIKE:

YOUR FAVOURITE GAMES AND TOYS ARE:

YOUR FAVOURITE SONGS AND RHYMES ARE:

YOUR FAVOURITE STORIES ARE:

YOUR FAVOURITE THINGS ARE:

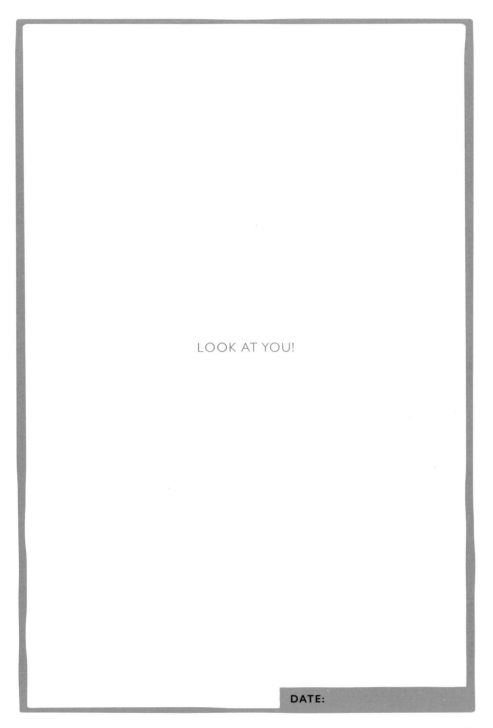

LOOK AT YOU!

DATE:

'ANY-DAY' RECORDS AND PHOTOS

AGE:

DATE:

YOU WAKE UP AT:

YOU GET UP AT:

YOU HAVE A NAP AT:

YOUR BEDTIME IS:

YOU ARE FED AT:

MINI MILESTONES:

YOU LIKE:

YOU DON'T LIKE:

YOUR FAVOURITE GAMES AND TOYS ARE:

YOUR FAVOURITE SONGS AND RHYMES ARE:

YOUR FAVOURITE STORIES ARE:

YOUR FAVOURITE THINGS ARE:

AGE:

DATE:

YOU WAKE UP AT:

YOU GET UP AT:

YOU HAVE A NAP AT:

YOUR BEDTIME IS:

YOU ARE FED AT:

MINI MILESTONES:

YOU LIKE:

YOU DON'T LIKE:

YOUR FAVOURITE GAMES AND TOYS ARE:

YOUR FAVOURITE SONGS AND RHYMES ARE:

YOUR FAVOURITE STORIES ARE:

YOUR FAVOURITE THINGS ARE:

'ANY-DAY' RECORDS AND PHOTOS

AGE:

DATE:

YOU WAKE UP AT:

YOU GET UP AT:

YOU HAVE A NAP AT:

YOUR BEDTIME IS:

YOU ARE FED AT:

MINI MILESTONES:

YOU LIKE:

YOU DON'T LIKE:

YOUR FAVOURITE GAMES AND TOYS ARE:

YOUR FAVOURITE SONGS AND RHYMES ARE:

YOUR FAVOURITE STORIES ARE:

YOUR FAVOURITE THINGS ARE:

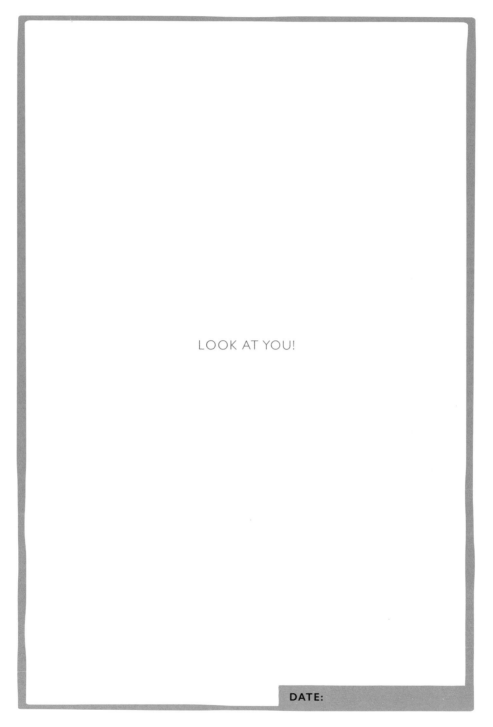

LOOK AT YOU!

DATE:

'ANY-DAY' RECORDS AND PHOTOS

AGE:

DATE:

YOU WAKE UP AT:

YOU GET UP AT:

YOU HAVE A NAP AT:

YOUR BEDTIME IS:

YOU ARE FED AT:

MINI MILESTONES:

YOU LIKE:

YOU DON'T LIKE:

YOUR FAVOURITE GAMES AND TOYS ARE:

YOUR FAVOURITE SONGS AND RHYMES ARE:

YOUR FAVOURITE STORIES ARE:

YOUR FAVOURITE THINGS ARE:

AGE: ....

DATE: ....

YOU WAKE UP AT: ....

YOU GET UP AT: ....

YOU HAVE A NAP AT: ....

YOUR BEDTIME IS: ....

YOU ARE FED AT: ....

MINI MILESTONES: ....

....

....

YOU LIKE: ....

....

YOU DON'T LIKE: ....

....

YOUR FAVOURITE GAMES AND TOYS ARE: ....

....

....

YOUR FAVOURITE SONGS AND RHYMES ARE: ....

....

....

YOUR FAVOURITE STORIES ARE: ....

....

....

....

YOUR FAVOURITE THINGS ARE: ....

....

....

....

'ANY-DAY' RECORDS AND PHOTOS

AGE:

DATE:

YOU WAKE UP AT:

YOU GET UP AT:

YOU HAVE A NAP AT:

YOUR BEDTIME IS:

YOU ARE FED AT:

MINI MILESTONES:

YOU LIKE:

YOU DON'T LIKE:

YOUR FAVOURITE GAMES AND TOYS ARE:

YOUR FAVOURITE SONGS AND RHYMES ARE:

YOUR FAVOURITE STORIES ARE:

YOUR FAVOURITE THINGS ARE:

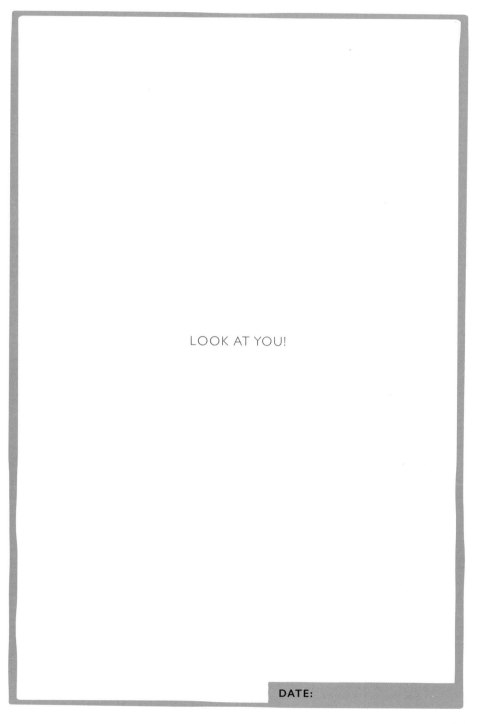

LOOK AT YOU!

DATE:

PLACES YOU LIKE TO VISIT

FAVOURITE PARKS, FAVOURED AUNTIES –
WHERE DO YOU LIKE BEST TO GO?

DATE:

Making friends and learning to play together is a part of growing up. Record your baby's early friendships in words and pictures.

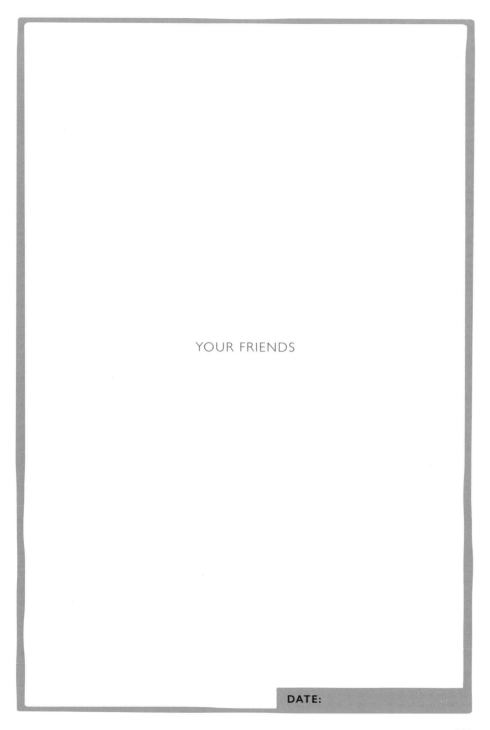

YOUR FRIENDS

DATE:

THINGS WE LIKE TO DO TOGETHER

As your baby grows and their interest in the world is sparked, you'll enjoy taking part in more and more activities together. Whether its music or dancing classes, going to the park, feeding the ducks, a baby group, or making cakes, make a record of what you both enjoy about it here.

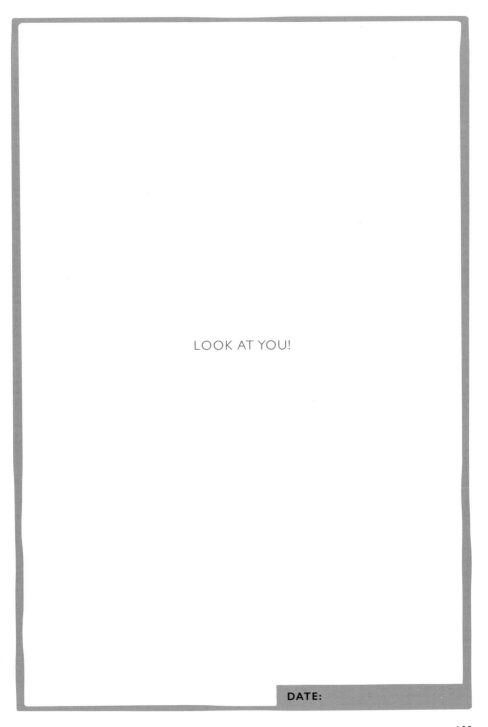

LOOK AT YOU!

DATE:

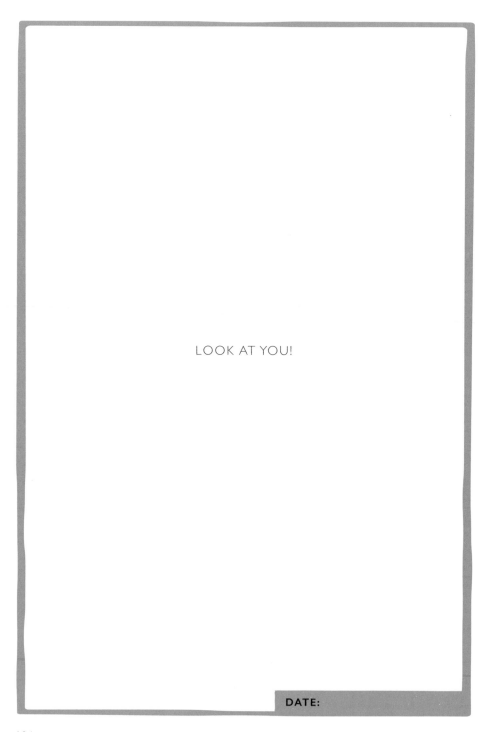

LOOK AT YOU!

DATE:

THINGS WE LIKE TO DO TOGETHER

MESSY MEALTIMES

Now that your baby is eating regular meals, why not make a note of their favourite foods, as well as recording some memories of those occasions when things got a bit messy!

YOUR FAVOURITE BREAKFAST IS:

....
....
....

YOUR FAVOURITE SNACK IS:

....
....
....

AT LUNCHTIME YOU LIKE TO EAT:

....
....
....

AT DINNER TIME YOU ENJOY:

....
....
....

A FUNNY MEMORY:

....
....
....
....
....
....
....

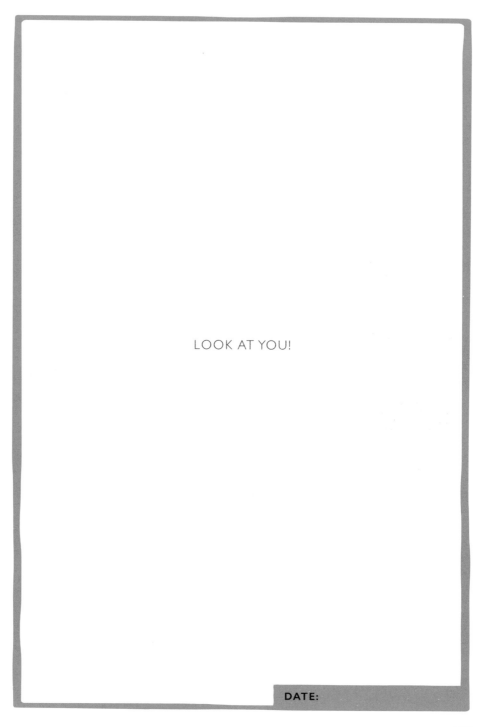

LOOK AT YOU!

DATE:

YOUR BEDTIME ROUTINE

YOU GO TO SLEEP AT:

....

....

BEFORE YOU GO TO SLEEP YOU LIKE:

....

....

....

....

....

....

....

....

YOUR FAVOURITE LULLABIES AND BOOKS AT BEDTIME ARE:

....

....

....

....

....

....

....

OTHER COMMENTS:

....

....

....

....

....

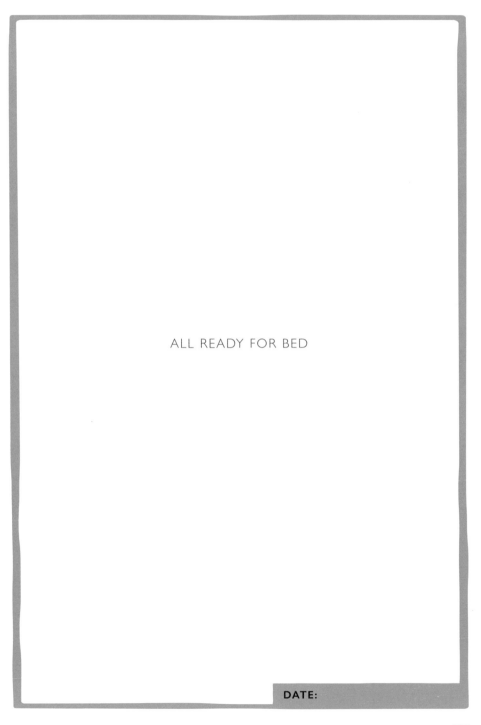

ALL READY FOR BED

DATE:

REFLECTIONS

It's easy to get lost in the busyness of everyday living, so why not take some time to reflect back over the past months together; your favourite moments and your difficult times too. Record what you have learned about yourself and each other, as well as your baby.

YOUR SECOND CHRISTMAS

AGE:
....

WE SPENT CHRISTMAS EVE AT:
....

WITH:
....

....

WE SPENT CHRISTMAS DAY AT:
....

WITH:
....

....

YOUR CHRISTMAS OUTFIT WAS:
....

....

YOU ATE:
....

....

YOU RECEIVED LOTS OF PRESENTS INCLUDING:
....

....

....

YOU ENJOYED:
....

....

....

....

....

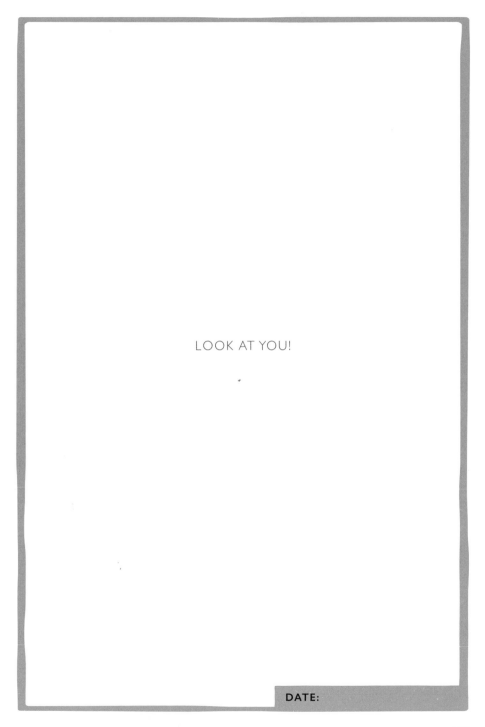

LOOK AT YOU!

DATE:

OCCASIONS TO REMEMBER

Every year has memorable events, from family weddings and births to christenings or naming ceremonies. Use these pages to record what was celebrated when, who was there and what was special about it.

OCCASION:
....
....

DATE:
....

WHO WAS THERE:
....
....
....
....
....

MEMORIES OF THE DAY:
....
....
....
....
....
....
....
....
....
....
....

OCCASION:

....

....

....

DATE:

....

WHO WAS THERE:

....

....

....

....

....

....

MEMORIES OF THE DAY:

....

....

....

....

....

....

....

....

....

....

....

OCCASIONS TO REMEMBER

OCCASION:

DATE:

WHO WAS THERE:

MEMORIES OF THE DAY:

OCCASION:

DATE:

WHO WAS THERE:

MEMORIES OF THE DAY:

HOLIDAYS

AGE:

WE WENT TO:

ON:

FOR:

YOUR FAVOURITE THING ABOUT THE HOLIDAY WAS:

YOU LIKED:

YOU DIDN'T LIKE:

REFLECTIONS:

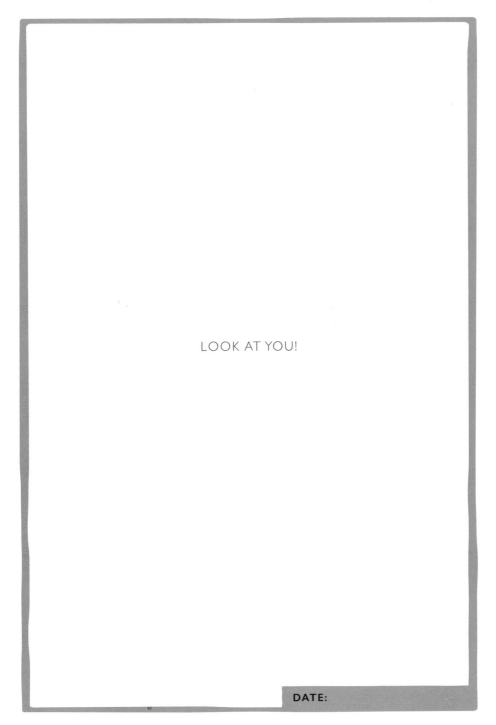

LOOK AT YOU!

DATE:

YOUR SECOND BIRTHDAY

WAS SPENT AT:

YOU WERE GIVEN:

YOUR CAKE WAS:

ON YOUR BIRTHDAY WE:

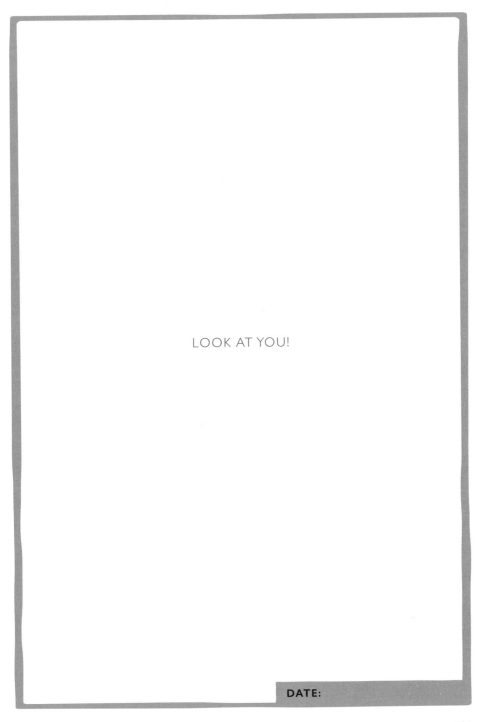

LOOK AT YOU!

DATE:

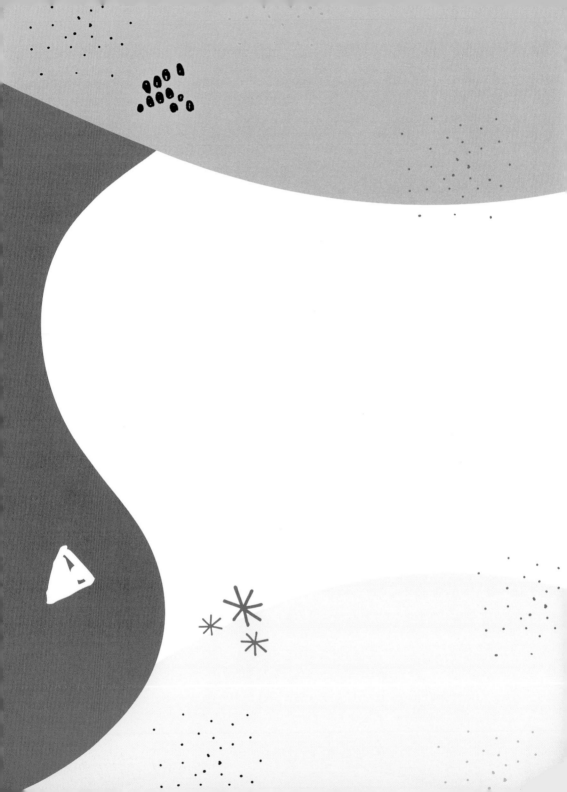

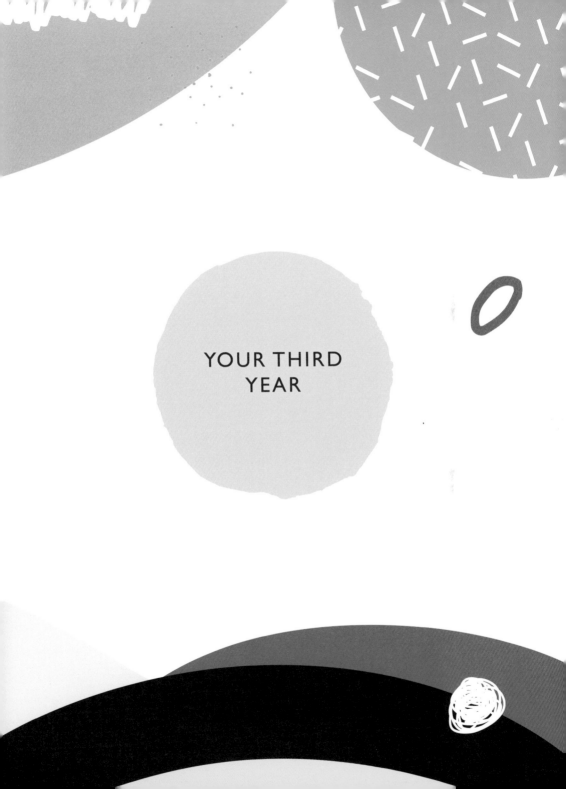

YOUR THIRD
YEAR

NOW YOU ARE TWO ...

YOU ARE: CMS/INS TALL

YOU WEIGH: KGS/LBS

YOU CAN:

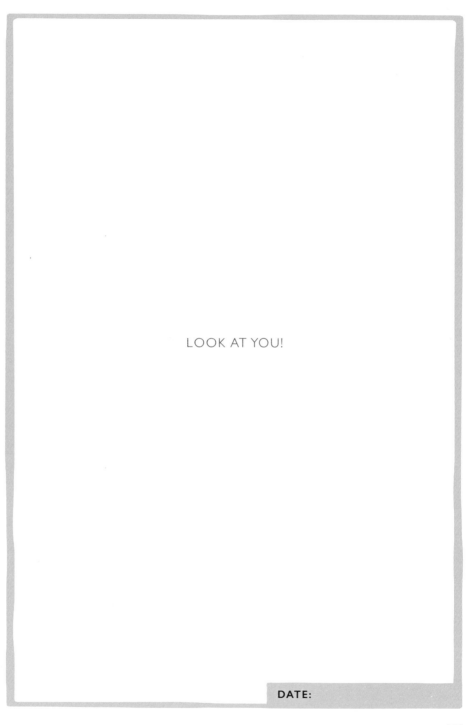

LOOK AT YOU!

DATE:

'ANY-DAY' RECORDS AND PHOTOS

AGE:

DATE:

YOU WAKE UP AT:

YOU GET UP AT:

YOU HAVE A NAP AT:

YOUR BEDTIME IS:

YOU ARE FED AT:

MINI MILESTONES:

YOU LIKE:

YOU DON'T LIKE:

YOUR FAVOURITE GAMES AND TOYS ARE:

YOUR FAVOURITE SONGS AND RHYMES ARE:

YOUR FAVOURITE STORIES ARE:

YOUR FAVOURITE THINGS ARE:

AGE:

DATE:

YOU WAKE UP AT:

YOU GET UP AT:

YOU HAVE A NAP AT:

YOUR BEDTIME IS:

YOU ARE FED AT:

MINI MILESTONES:

YOU LIKE:

YOU DON'T LIKE:

YOUR FAVOURITE GAMES AND TOYS ARE:

YOUR FAVOURITE SONGS AND RHYMES ARE:

YOUR FAVOURITE STORIES ARE:

YOUR FAVOURITE THINGS ARE:

'ANY-DAY' RECORDS AND PHOTOS

AGE:

DATE:

YOU WAKE UP AT:

YOU GET UP AT:

YOU HAVE A NAP AT:

YOUR BEDTIME IS:

YOU ARE FED AT:

MINI MILESTONES:

YOU LIKE:

YOU DON'T LIKE:

YOUR FAVOURITE GAMES AND TOYS ARE:

YOUR FAVOURITE SONGS AND RHYMES ARE:

YOUR FAVOURITE STORIES ARE:

YOUR FAVOURITE THINGS ARE:

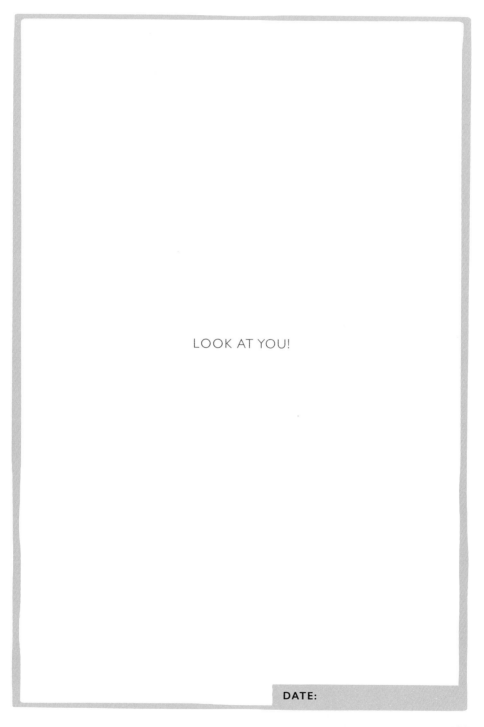

LOOK AT YOU!

'ANY-DAY' RECORDS AND PHOTOS

AGE:

DATE:

YOU WAKE UP AT:

YOU GET UP AT:

YOU HAVE A NAP AT:

YOUR BEDTIME IS:

YOU ARE FED AT:

MINI MILESTONES:

YOU LIKE:

YOU DON'T LIKE:

YOUR FAVOURITE GAMES AND TOYS ARE:

YOUR FAVOURITE SONGS AND RHYMES ARE:

YOUR FAVOURITE STORIES ARE:

YOUR FAVOURITE THINGS ARE:

AGE:

DATE:

YOU WAKE UP AT:

YOU GET UP AT:

YOU HAVE A NAP AT:

YOUR BEDTIME IS:

YOU ARE FED AT:

MINI MILESTONES:

YOU LIKE:

YOU DON'T LIKE:

YOUR FAVOURITE GAMES AND TOYS ARE:

YOUR FAVOURITE SONGS AND RHYMES ARE:

YOUR FAVOURITE STORIES ARE:

YOUR FAVOURITE THINGS ARE:

'ANY-DAY' RECORDS AND PHOTOS

AGE:

DATE:

YOU WAKE UP AT:

YOU GET UP AT:

YOU HAVE A NAP AT:

YOUR BEDTIME IS:

YOU ARE FED AT:

MINI MILESTONES:

YOU LIKE:

YOU DON'T LIKE:

YOUR FAVOURITE GAMES AND TOYS ARE:

YOUR FAVOURITE SONGS AND RHYMES ARE:

YOUR FAVOURITE STORIES ARE:

YOUR FAVOURITE THINGS ARE:

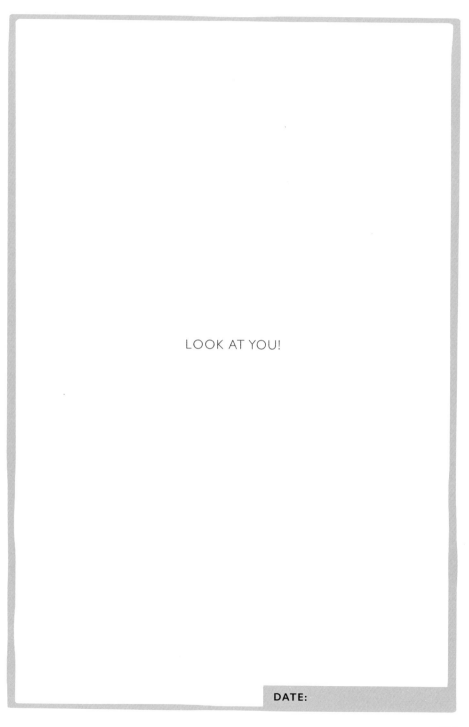

LOOK AT YOU!

DATE:

AGE:

DATE:

YOU WAKE UP AT:

YOU GET UP AT:

YOU HAVE A NAP AT:

YOUR BEDTIME IS:

YOU ARE FED AT:

MINI MILESTONES:

YOU LIKE:

YOU DON'T LIKE:

YOUR FAVOURITE GAMES AND TOYS ARE:

YOUR FAVOURITE SONGS AND RHYMES ARE:

YOUR FAVOURITE STORIES ARE:

YOUR FAVOURITE THINGS ARE:

AGE: ....

DATE: ....

YOU WAKE UP AT: ....

YOU GET UP AT: ....

YOU HAVE A NAP AT: ....

YOUR BEDTIME IS: ....

YOU ARE FED AT: ....

MINI MILESTONES: ....

....

....

YOU LIKE: ....

....

YOU DON'T LIKE: ....

....

YOUR FAVOURITE GAMES AND TOYS ARE: ....

....

....

YOUR FAVOURITE SONGS AND RHYMES ARE: ....

....

....

YOUR FAVOURITE STORIES ARE: ....

....

....

....

YOUR FAVOURITE THINGS ARE: ....

....

....

....

AGE:

DATE:

YOU WAKE UP AT:

YOU GET UP AT:

YOU HAVE A NAP AT:

YOUR BEDTIME IS:

YOU ARE FED AT:

MINI MILESTONES:

YOU LIKE:

YOU DON'T LIKE:

YOUR FAVOURITE GAMES AND TOYS ARE:

YOUR FAVOURITE SONGS AND RHYMES ARE:

YOUR FAVOURITE STORIES ARE:

YOUR FAVOURITE THINGS ARE:

LOOK AT YOU!

PLACES YOU LIKE TO VISIT

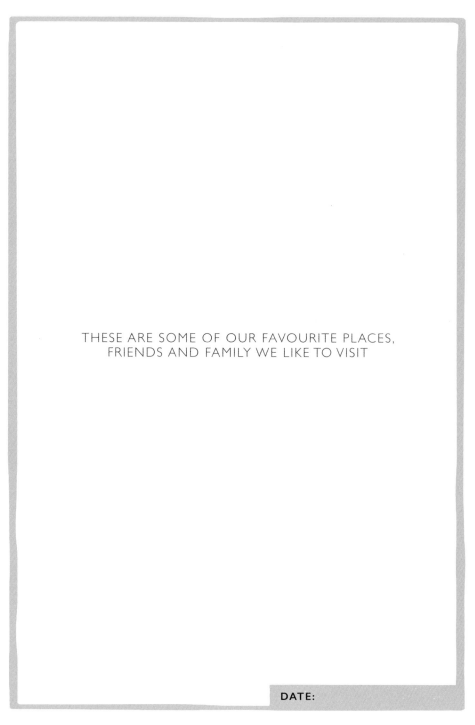

THESE ARE SOME OF OUR FAVOURITE PLACES,
FRIENDS AND FAMILY WE LIKE TO VISIT

DATE:

YOUR BEST FRIENDS ARE:

....
....
....
....
....
....
....
....
....
....
....

GAMES YOU LIKE TO PLAY:

....
....
....
....
....
....
....
....
....
....
....
....
....

AS YOUR BABY'S CIRCLE WIDENS,
FRIENDSHIPS WILL BLOSSOM.
TAKE A PHOTO OF BEST FRIENDS TOGETHER.

DATE:

YOUR FRIENDS

YOUR BEST FRIENDS ARE:

....
....
....
....
....
....
....
....
....
....
....

GAMES YOU LIKE TO PLAY:

....
....
....
....
....
....
....
....
....
....
....
....

THINGS WE LIKE TO DO TOGETHER

What do you and your baby like to do together? Do you have favourite songs or games? Perhaps you like to go to the park or swimming. It's often the everyday activities that we forget so easily, but these are the activities that forge our relationship and which shape your baby's life, so record them here to share together later.

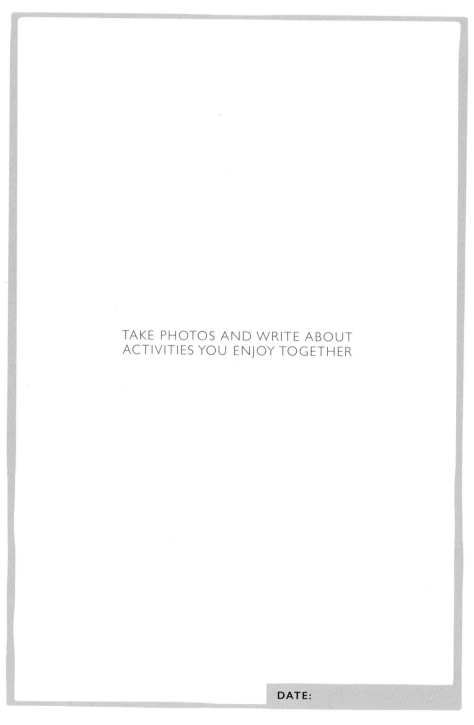

TAKE PHOTOS AND WRITE ABOUT
ACTIVITIES YOU ENJOY TOGETHER

DATE:

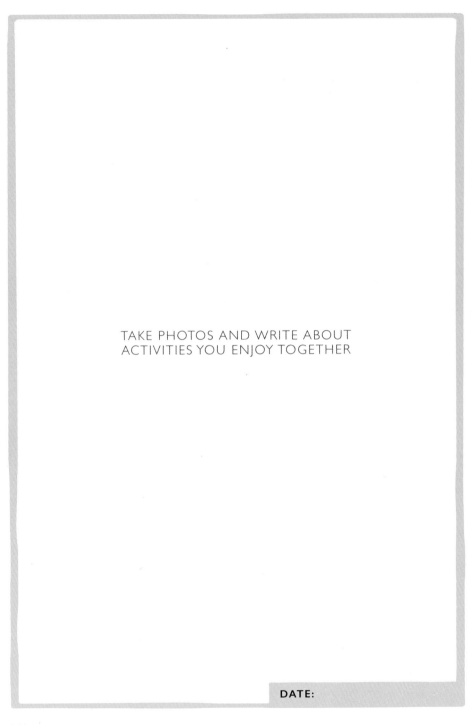

TAKE PHOTOS AND WRITE ABOUT
ACTIVITIES YOU ENJOY TOGETHER

DATE:

THINGS WE LIKE TO DO TOGETHER

REFLECTIONS

It's easy to get lost in the busyness of everyday living, so why not take some time to reflect back over these first months together; your favourite moments and your difficult times too. Record what you have learned about yourself and each other, as well as your baby.

YOUR FAVOURITE RECIPES

It can be great fun finding new foods for your baby to try. Record some of their favourite recipes here; write down the ingredients, how you made them and any memories of favourite meals.

INGREDIENTS: METHOD:

MEALTIME MEMORIES:

INGREDIENTS:

METHOD:

MEALTIME MEMORIES:

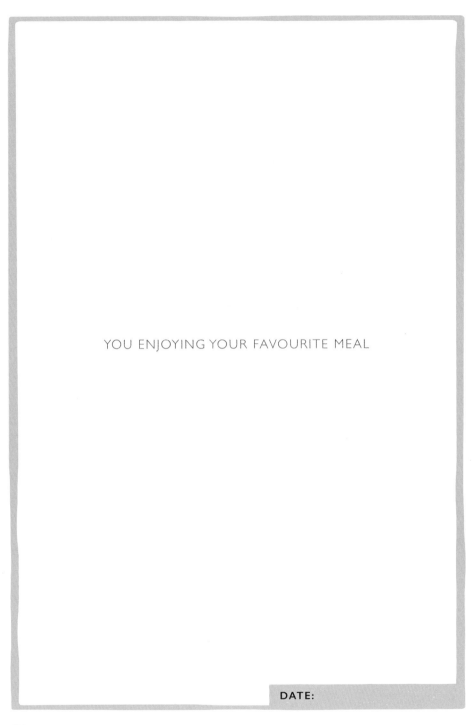

YOU ENJOYING YOUR FAVOURITE MEAL

DATE:

YOUR FAVOURITE RECIPES

INGREDIENTS: METHOD:

MEALTIME MEMORIES:

YOUR BEDTIME ROUTINE

YOU GO TO SLEEP AT:

BEFORE YOU GO TO SLEEP YOU LIKE:

YOUR FAVOURITE LULLABIES AND BOOKS AT BEDTIME ARE:

OTHER COMMENTS:

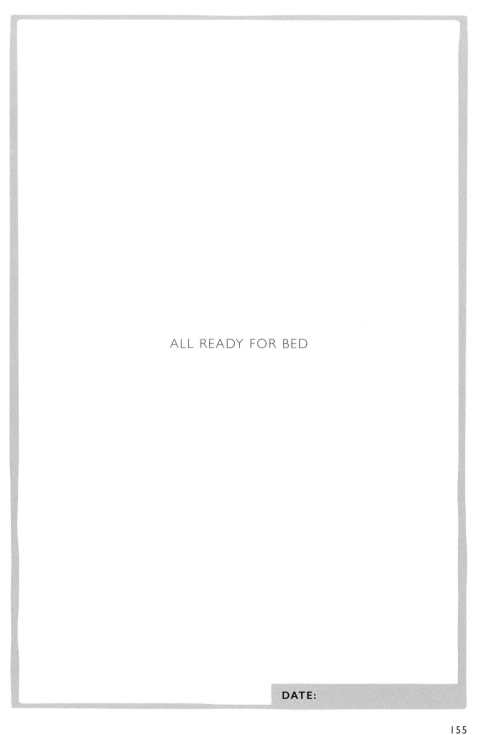

ALL READY FOR BED

DATE:

YOUR THIRD CHRISTMAS

AGE:

WE SPENT CHRISTMAS EVE AT:

WITH:

WE SPENT CHRISTMAS DAY AT:

WITH:

YOUR CHRISTMAS OUTFIT WAS:

YOU ATE:

YOU RECEIVED LOTS OF PRESENTS INCLUDING:

YOU ENJOYED:

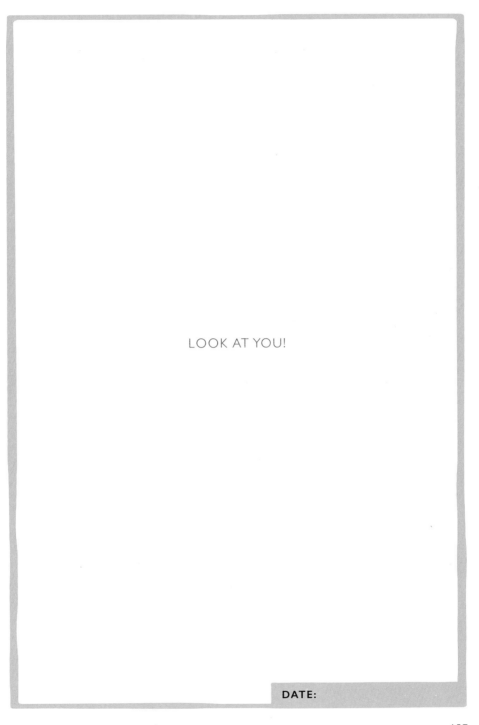

LOOK AT YOU!

DATE:

OCCASIONS TO REMEMBER

Every year has memorable events, from family weddings and births to christenings or naming ceremonies. Use these pages to record what was celebrated when, who was there and what was special about it.

OCCASION:

DATE:

WHO WAS THERE:

MEMORIES OF THE DAY:

OCCASION:

DATE:

WHO WAS THERE:

MEMORIES OF THE DAY:

OCCASIONS TO REMEMBER

OCCASION:

DATE:

WHO WAS THERE:

MEMORIES OF THE DAY:

OCCASION:

....

....

....

DATE:

....

WHO WAS THERE:

....

....

....

....

....

....

....

MEMORIES OF THE DAY:

....

....

....

....

....

....

....

....

....

....

....

HOLIDAYS

AGE:

WE WENT TO:

ON:

FOR:

YOUR FAVOURITE THING ABOUT THE HOLIDAY WAS:

YOU LIKED:

YOU DIDN'T LIKE:

REFLECTIONS:

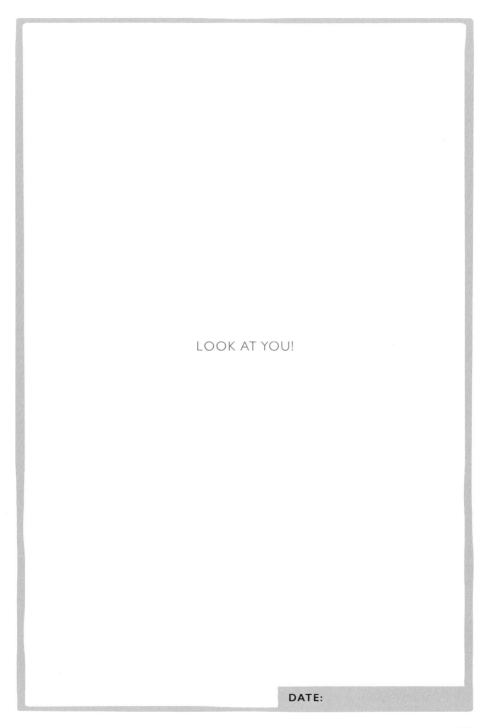

LOOK AT YOU!

DATE:

YOUR THIRD BIRTHDAY

WAS SPENT AT:

YOU WERE GIVEN:

YOUR CAKE WAS:

ON YOUR BIRTHDAY WE:

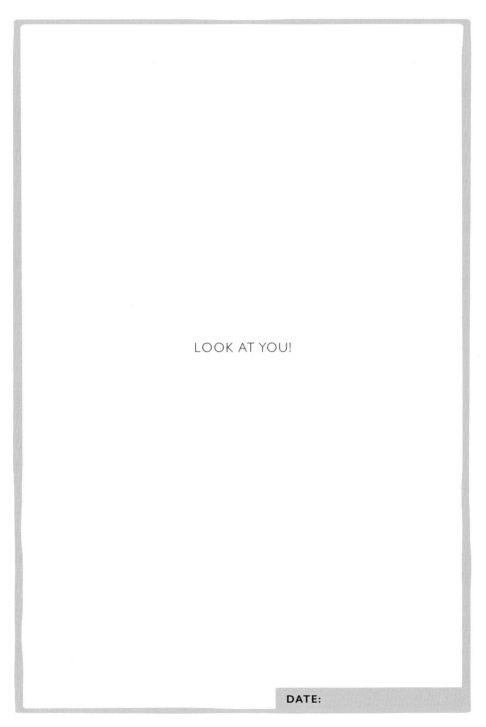

LOOK AT YOU!

DATE:

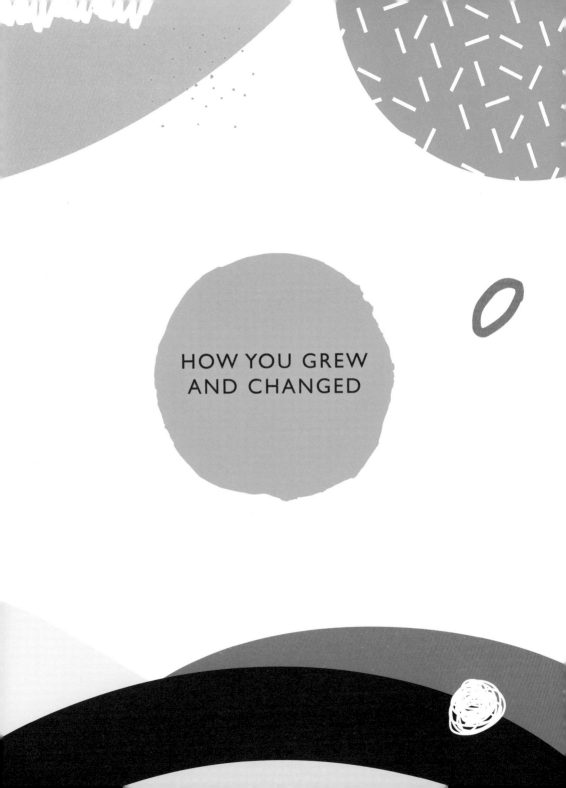

HOW YOU GREW
AND CHANGED

YOUR DEVELOPMENT

AGE	WEIGHT	LENGTH
BIRTH		
I WEEK		
2 WEEKS		
3 WEEKS		
4 WEEKS		
5 WEEKS		
6 WEEKS		
7 WEEKS		
8 WEEKS		
9 WEEKS		
10 WEEKS		
11 WEEKS		
12 WEEKS		

EYE COLOUR	HAIR COLOUR/TYPE

YOUR DEVELOPMENT

AGE	WEIGHT	LENGTH
4 MONTHS		
5 MONTHS		
6 MONTHS		
7 MONTHS		
8 MONTHS		
9 MONTHS		
10 MONTHS		
11 MONTHS		
1 YEAR		
18 MONTHS		
2 YEARS		
2½ YEARS		
3 YEARS		

EYE COLOUR	HAIR COLOUR/TYPE

YOUR HEALTH

YOUR DOCTOR'S NAME IS:

YOUR BLOOD GROUP IS:

YOU ARE ALLERGIC TO:

YOU WERE ILL WITH:

DATE:

DATE:

DATE:

DATE:

DATE:

DATE:

DATE:

DATE:

DATE:

DATE:

DATE:

DATE:

DATE:

DATE:

DATE:

DATE:

DATE:

DATE:

DATE:

VACCINE	DATE	AGE	REACTION

Make a note of the date each tooth comes in.

UPPER

1.   6.

2.   7.

3.   8.

4.   9.

5.   10.

LOWER

1.   6.

2.   7.

3.   8.

4.   9.

5.   10.

WE KNEW YOU WERE TEETHING WHEN:

YOUR FIRST TOOTH

DATE:

YOU LEARNT TO LIFT YOUR HEAD DURING TUMMY TIME

DATE:

YOU HELD A TOY

DATE:

YOU ROLLED OVER

DATE:

YOU SAT UP BY YOURSELF

DATE:

BEFORE YOU LEARN TO WALK...
YOU PULL YOURSELF ALONG

DATE:

...PERHAPS YOU LEARN TO CRAWL

DATE:

EVENTUALLY YOU PULL YOURSELF UP TO STANDING...

DATE:

...AND THEN WALKING IS EASY –
WITH A LITTLE HELP FROM YOUR FRIENDS

DATE:

Communication is about more than words. Babies communicate with their eyes, hands and the sounds they make. They often express emotion through their whole body. A mother can often tell what is wrong with her baby just by listening to the tone of their cry.... Share the ways you and your baby communicate with each other below.

SIGNS YOU USE TO TELL US THINGS:

FIRST WORDS:

THINGS YOU SAY THAT MAKE US LAUGH:

LOOK WHAT YOU'VE DRAWN!

DATE:

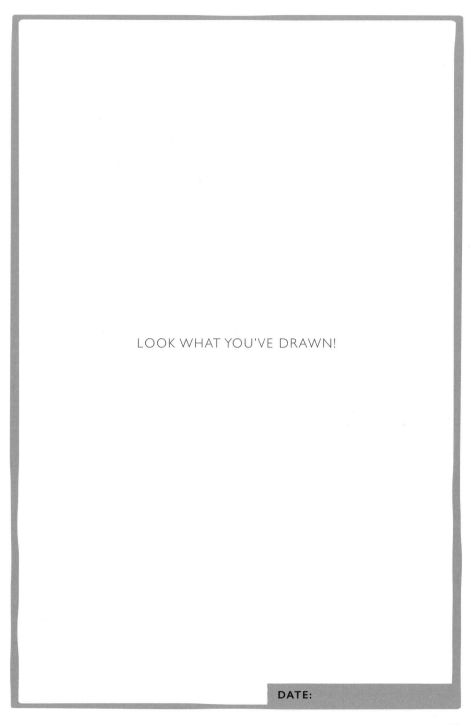

LOOK WHAT YOU'VE DRAWN!

DATE:

LOOK WHAT YOU'VE DRAWN!

DATE:

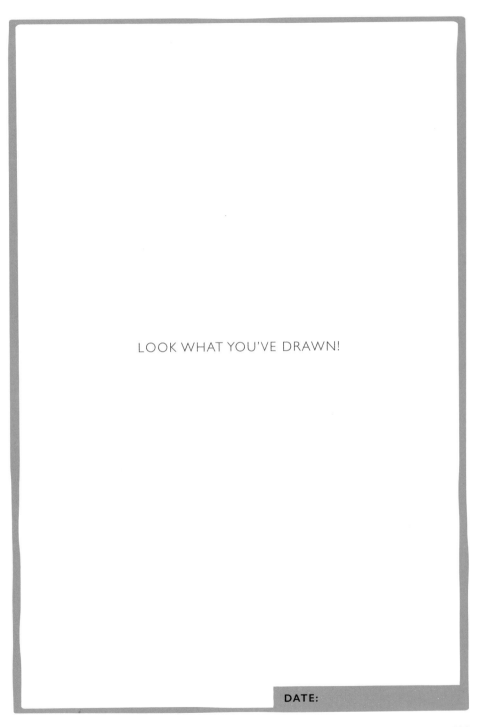

LOOK WHAT YOU'VE DRAWN!

DATE:

EVERY BABY GETS INTO MISCHIEF –
OFTEN PROVIDING WONDERFUL
PHOTO OPPORTUNITIES

DATE:

YOUR FIRST DAY AT NURSERY

YOUR NURSERY IS:

YOUR KEY WORKER IS:

YOUR HELPERS ARE:

YOUR FRIENDS ARE:

YOU LIKE TO:

YOU DON'T LIKE TO:

REFLECTIONS ON THE DAY:

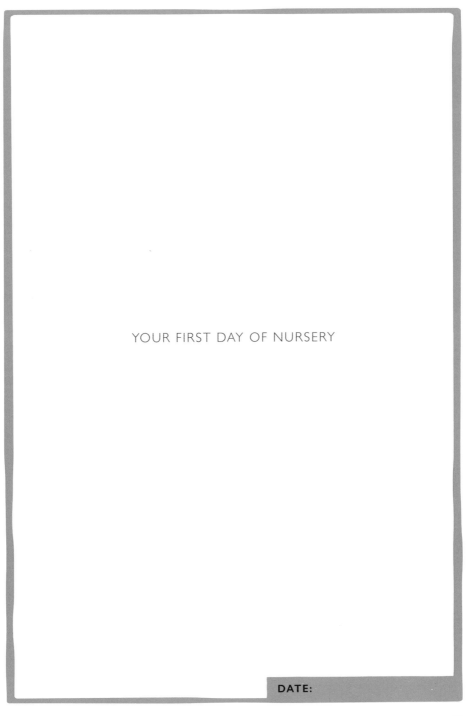

YOUR FIRST DAY OF NURSERY

DATE:

YOUR UNIQUE FIRSTS

The significance of when your baby first does something will vary from family to family. This page is an opportunity for you to record the other firsts ... firsts that have particular meaning for you – first smile, first kisses, first haircut, first time swimming, first time sleeping through the night, first time using a potty ... whatever special event you would like to mark.

EVENT	DATE	COMMENTS

EVENT	DATE	COMMENTS

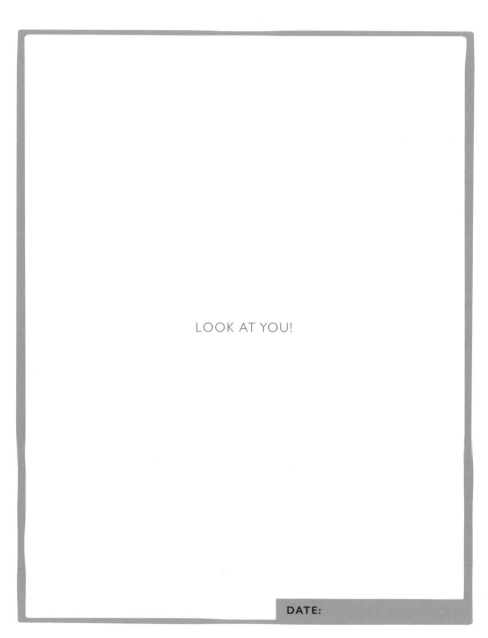

LOOK AT YOU!

DATE:

EVENT	DATE	COMMENTS

WHEN YOUR BABY IS SMALL,
WHY NOT TAKE THEIR PHOTO IN THE
SAME CHAIR OR LOCATION OVER A PERIOD
OF MONTHS. THEN YOU WILL SEE HOW
MUCH THEY ARE GROWING.

DATE:

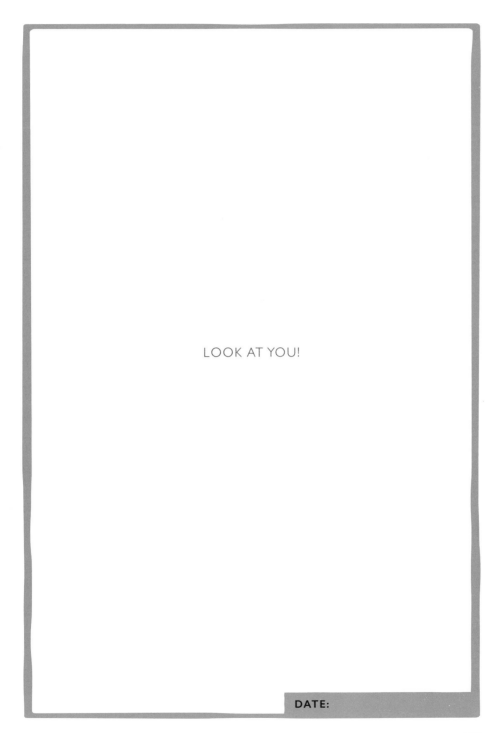

LOOK AT YOU!

DATE:

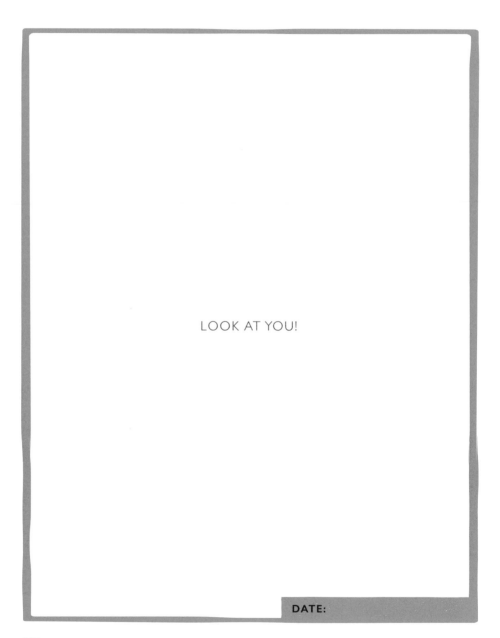

LOOK AT YOU!

DATE:

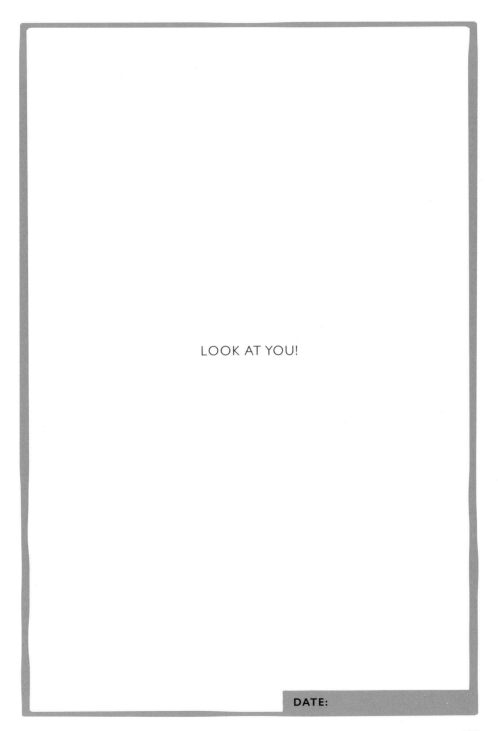

LOOK AT YOU!

DATE:

LOOKING BACK...

REFLECTIONS:

WHAT YOU WANTED US TO WRITE ABOUT HERE:

These are some of the things that your family members remember about your birth and your early years, as well as the special things they want to say to you.

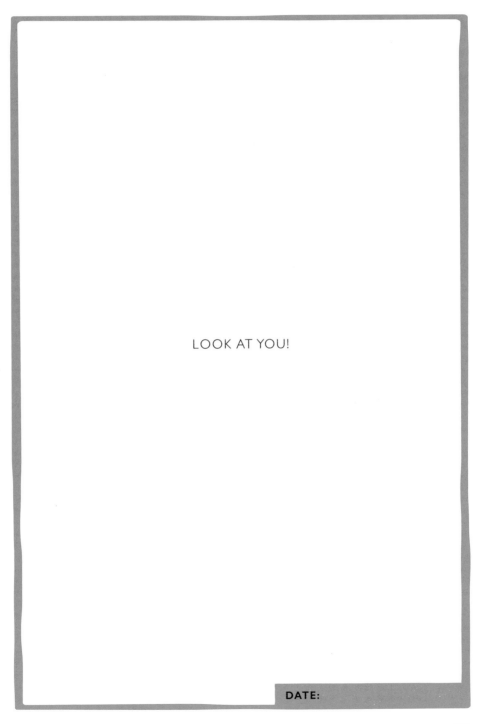

LOOK AT YOU!

DATE:

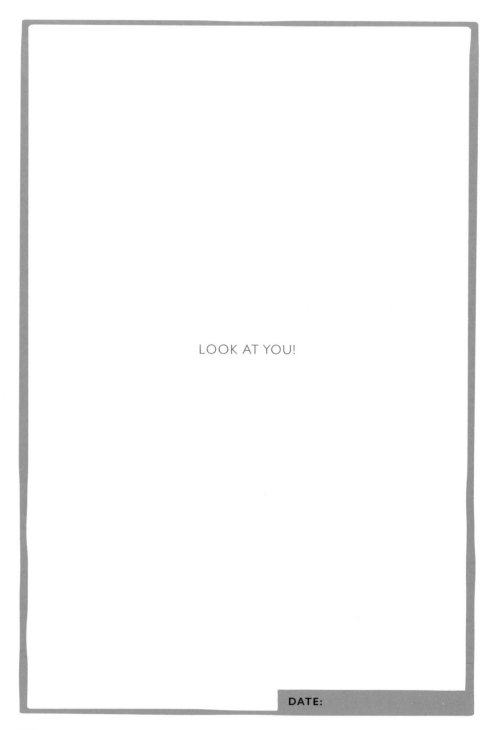

LOOK AT YOU!

DATE:

MESSAGES FROM YOUR FAMILY

MESSAGES FROM YOUR FAMILY

LOOK AT YOU!

DATE:

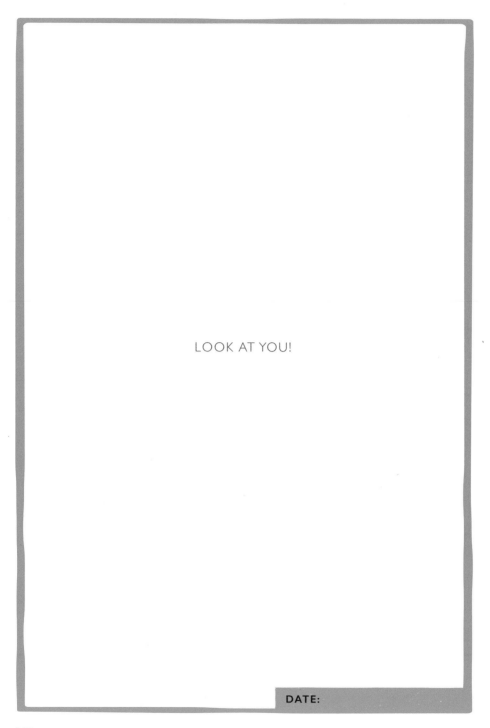

LOOK AT YOU!

DATE:

MESSAGES FROM YOUR FAMILY

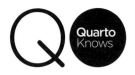

Brimming with creative inspiration, how-to projects and useful information to enrich your everyday life, Quarto Knows is a favourite destination for those pursuing their interests and passions. Visit our site and dig deeper with our books into your area of interest: Quarto Creates, Quarto Cooks, Quarto Homes, Quarto Lives, Quarto Drives, Quarto Explores, Quarto Gifts, or Quarto Kids.

Baby Book
© 2020 Quarto Publishing plc
Cover & interior illustrations © MURRIRA/Shutterstock.com

First published in 2020 by Frances Lincoln,
an imprint of The Quarto Group.
The Old Brewery, 6 Blundell Street
London, N7 9BH,
United Kingdom
T (0)20 7700 6700
www.QuartoKnows.com

Every effort has been made to trace the copyright holders of material quoted in this book.
If application is made in writing to the publisher, any omissions will be included in future editions.

A catalogue record for this book is available from the British Library.

ISBN 978 0 7112 5371 1

10 9 8 7 6 5 4 3 2 1

Design by Sarah Pyke

Printed in Singapore

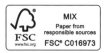